THE ESSENTIAL PATIENT HANDBOOK

THE ESSENTIAL PATIENT HANDBOOK:

Getting the Health Care You Need – From Doctors Who Know

ALAN B. ETTINGER, M.D.

AND

DEBORAH M. WEISBROT, M.D.

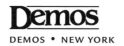

DEMOS • NEW YORK

"Drs. Ettinger and Weisbrot have compiled an exhaustive, educational primer for patients and their families... *The Essential Patient Handbook* provides a critically needed foundation for patient-centered, high quality medical care." *Arthur A. Levin M.P.H., Director, Center for Medical Consumers*

"*The Essential Patient Handbook* is not just a book you should have in case you should happen to be a patient one day (which we all will be!), but it is an essential home reference. A reference every family will use and, in fact, use often!" *John J. Connolly, Ed.D., Castle Connolly Top Doctors Guides*

"If you're like most people, navigating through the portals of modern medicine and the maze of conflicting health information in the media can be very confusing—even dangerous. How do you know if the health information you're receiving is accurate or not? Where can you turn to find out? Who can you trust to provide reliable guidance?... This first-of-its-kind resource provides invaluable insight that helps educate readers in becoming better, more informed consumers in the healthcare decision-making process.... *The Essential Patient Handbook* is 'hands-down' the most informative book on the market for those genuinely interested in taking charge of their own personal health and wellness journey." *Teresa Tanoos, News Anchor and Medical Reporter, "Healthy Living with Teresa Tanoos"*

"In today's healthcare world it is critical that patients take an active role in their medical care process. This book provides vital information to ensure that patients are informed, prepared and empowered." *Roxanne Black, Founder and Executive Director of Friends' Health Connection*

"When asked 'How long will doctors keep playing God?' Dr. William Osler, the doyen of U.S. medical education responded, 'When the patients get off of their knees.' *The Essential Patient Handbook* is of invaluable assistance in supporting patients, and their families in assuming this new upright position... The ideal doctor-patient relationship exists as a true partnership; this novel handbook provides the most essential, real-life scenarios on attaining that." *Rick Rader, M.D., Editor in Chief, Exceptional Parent Magazine*

"Having strong communication between the health care team and the patient and family can make a big difference in the care a patient receives. Kudos to Dr. Alan Ettinger and Dr. Deborah Weisbrot on helping patients know what to ask and how to ask it." *John Davis, CEO, National Kidney Foundation, Inc.*

"I would highly recommend this book for any patient who wants to take some responsibility for their own health care. *The Essential Patient Handbook* depicts simply how you can help yourself to better health care." *Seymour Diamond, M.D., Executive Chairman, National Headache Foundation; Director, Diamond Headache Clinic*

"It is an ideal text for patients who must deal with the complexities of today's medical system. The book is literally a roadmap that can direct a patient from point A to point Z. Without this roadmap a patient can wander through a labyrinth of twists and turns and find no resolution. Even more to the point it encourages patients to come armed for battle when they face the bewildering choices they must make to survive." *Dr. Frank Field, Meteorologist and Host of the television show "Research Update"*

"Drs. Ettinger and Weisbrot have produced a wonderful book on empowering patients and improving the physician-patient relationship. It helps patients become actively engaged in their care by helping them make judgments about prevention and treatment… Congratulations on tackling such an essential issue." *Michael Dowling, President and CEO of the North Shore-Long Island Jewish Health System*

"…demystifies the doctor patient interaction and can help in the development of a more meaningful relationship between a fully informed and prepared patient and consequently, a potentially more receptive physician." *John Barry, M.D., Clinical Associate Professor of Psychiatry, Stanford University Medical Center*

Demos Medical Publishing, 386 Park Avenue South,
New York, NY 10016

Visit our website at www.demosmedpub.com

Cover photo by Ronald J. Krowne

Book design and composition by Valerie Brewster,
Scribe Typography

Library of Congress Cataloging-in-Publication Data

Ettinger, Alan B.
The essential patient handbook: getting the health care
you need from doctors who know / Alan B. Ettinger and
Deborah M. Weisbrot.
    p.   cm.
Includes bibliographical references and index.
ISBN 1-932603-02-6 (alk. paper)
1. Physician and patient—Handbooks, manuals, etc.
2. Patients—Handbooks, manuals, etc.   3. Ambulatory
medical care—Handbooks, manuals, etc.   I. Weisbrot,
Deborah M., 1954–   II. Title.
R727.3.E89 2004
610.69'6—dc22
                                        2004008479

To access the downloadable PDFs that come
with your purchase of this title please go to:

http://www.demosmedpub.com/essential.html

and use the word "demos" when prompted for
a password.

Dedication

To my brother David and father Samuel. Throughout our long struggle with medical illness, they have always been by our side.

A.E.

To my parents, Pauline and Aaron Weisbrot. I stand in awe of their extraordinary courage in the face of multiple medical problems. To my brother, Jeffrey and sister-in-law, Andrea, who have always been a great support to us.

D.W.

We would both like to dedicate this book to Dr. Marvin Don, the quintessential role model for a compassionate and caring physician.

Finally, we dedicate this book to our patients, who have given us the privilege of working with them and who have taught us so much through the years.

Acknowledgments

We would like to gratefully acknowledge the following friends and colleagues who invested countless hours reviewing assorted chapters in this book and who offered invaluable insights and suggestions:

Jenna Antonelli	Robert Kaplan
Ann Marie Bezuyen	Rich Libman
Diane Chrzanowski	Sheila Lobel
Orrin Devinsky	Alexandra Mcbride
Joel Don	Jessica Monas
David Ettinger	Gerry Novak
Mark Fauth	Rosie Olivares
Barry Florence	Laurie Ozelius
Joyce E. Fox	Jane Perr
Janice Gay	Linda Farber Post
Barbara Golden	Debbie Risbrook
Marjorie Gonzalez	Bernie Rosof
Angela Governale	Steven Schachter
Sandy Hamberger	Steve Schneider
Joanna Hamann	Angela Scicutella
Cynthia Holly	Candace Smith
Margaret Holmes	Robin Thompson
Ron Holmes	

We would also like to express our special thanks to our freelance book editor, Robert Kaplan of Robert Kaplan Associates, for his invaluable assistance in developing the manuscript for this book.

Table of Contents

Preface

With hundreds, perhaps thousands of books written for the public on health care, what can possibly be offered in a new book that has not been said before? If you are looking for a book describing one of the commonly encountered, pie-in-the-sky, idealized versions of the doctor-patient relationship or, alternatively, a book that bashes doctors or hospitals, then this book is not for you. This book is also not for you if you prefer to be passive and let the doctor do all the talking and tell you what to do without question. However, if you are one of the millions of Americans who are dissatisfied with their medical care and you are looking for a practical, no-nonsense way to get what you need from your doctors, this book definitely *is* for you. It will be a much-used companion in your search for optimal care.

The Essential Patient Handbook will take you through the entire medical evaluation process, from the first question to the last. It is a guide to the thorough preparation of your medical information *before* you see the doctor, and it will explain to you why each piece of information is crucial. The information you will learn to prepare with this book is symptom-specific and will help your doctor arrive at a differential diagnosis. Once a diagnosis is established, *The Handbook* will help you prepare everything else your doctors need to know in order to give you the best possible medical care. *The Handbook* includes many forms that will help you prepare in advance *all* of the information you need to share with your doctor *and* the questions you need to ask.

Why permit yourself to be intimidated, anxious, or flustered when you ask your doctor questions? *The Handbook* will arm you with the medical ammunition you need to fire off the essential questions you need to ask.

Finally, *The Handbook* will help you deal with the common problems that arise in doctor-patient interactions, including dealing with difficult doctors, analyzing your feelings about your doctor, talking to your doctor on the telephone, wading through the billing quagmire, surviving hospitalization, and discussing alternative medicine treatments. Having this knowledge will empower you to become partners with your doctors in achieving the most accurate diagnosis and best treatment. You can make the most of your visit to your doctor with these tools in hand.

Alan B. Ettinger, M.D.
Deborah M. Weisbrot, M.D.

Introduction by Deborah M. Weisbrot, M.D.

One winter day in 1995, I developed a bad cough and fever. As I was contacting my patients to reschedule their appointments, little did I know that I was about to embark on my own voyage of severe personal illness. This would prove to be one of the most terrifying and painful journeys I have ever endured, and one which I never could have previously imagined, even as a doctor.

Suddenly I found myself sitting in an emergency room, severely short of breath; yet no one seemed to recognize the extent of my distress. I waited for hours before being evaluated. I was sent home from the emergency room with a diagnosis of mild pneumonia; but I developed massive respiratory failure within 24 hours. Before long, I became completely paralyzed, unable to speak and connected to a respirator in order to breathe. I was transferred to a university hospital by ambulance where I was diagnosed with *Adult Respiratory Distress Syndrome* (ARDS). This is a disorder in which the lungs fill with fluid. I came very close to dying.

The next three months were a nightmare of pain and terror during which I was unable to communicate with those around me. As gowned and gloved staff rushed in and out of my room, attending to my medical needs, the majority seemed unaware that I was often conscious but unable to communicate. Only my husband and my family, who virtually lived at my bedside in the Intensive Care Unit (ICU), had any notion of what I was experiencing. Ironically, I was placed in the same ICU bed in which my husband had treated many of his sickest patients.

During my illness, I lost my identity as a doctor. No one ever called me by my professional name and I doubt most hospital staff knew that I was a doctor. What did it matter? I had been a healthy wife and mother of two little boys, but I woke up one winter day to find myself with a tube in my neck to breathe, unable to speak and unable to write due to paralysis. My baseline emotional state was one of extreme anxiety. I would fight going to sleep for fear that I would never wake up again, despite the fact that I was severely sleep deprived and desperately needed to sleep. I was intermittently delirious or confused. I experienced a waking dream in which I was trapped in a bed in the basement of a synagogue, struggling to get out, even trying to crawl. In the dream, a very compassionate woman was trying to help me, who I later recognized to be a wonderful nurse who was caring for me during the night shift.

From my ICU bed, where I stayed for months, I looked out the door and saw many healthy attending doctors and doctors-in-training. At times, I'd hear them laughing and joking. Of course, there was nothing wrong with that, but from my newly discovered patient's perspective, I felt that none of them had any idea what it felt like to be ill. Only a few special physicians directly expressed any empathy towards me in their interactions — the vast majority dealt with medical issues only. In contrast, many of the nursing and ancillary staff were quite compassionate; however, I also needed that type of interaction with the doctors caring for me. A simple comment or question such as, "You are really going through such an ordeal. What is it like for you?" would have meant a lot — even if I couldn't respond verbally.

From my doctor's perspective, I understood that the ICU physicians were caring for a group of desperately ill individuals and that they needed to focus on extremely complex medical problems. There is absolutely no question that the medical staff saved my life and I am extremely grateful for all their extraordinary efforts. I am also aware that they spent time explaining my medical condition to my family. Nonetheless, I also desperately needed the doctors to sit down at the bedside and acknowledge my struggle to survive in a more meaningful way. Against all odds, I did survive and, today, I walk into the very same hospital as a physician instead of a patient. Nine years later, hardly a day goes by that I don't look up to "my" window in the ICU and experience a surge of emotion when I think about my experiences there.

I had always considered myself to be an empathic physician, but I had to admit that only now did I truly understand how terrifying it can be to be a patient. Finally, I realized what it is like to be overwhelmed by a medical condition, to be helpless, and to be completely dependent upon others. My experience as a patient would probably have been worse if not for my physician-husband continuously advocating for me. Most patients are not fortunate enough to have such support. We hope that this book will help unravel the complexities of dealing with the doctor and will empower individuals to advocate for their needs.

I spent several years, and made innumerable doctor's office visits, recuperating from the effects of this devastating illness. Thanks to superb medical care, I survived with little residual lung damage. This experience of illness profoundly transformed my understanding of the difficulties my patients experience on a daily basis. From both sides of the hospital bed, I have come to realize the importance of communicating effectively and efficiently with doctors, preparing information to generate a complete history, and knowing what to expect in return. I now know how vitally important it is for doctors to listen to their patients and that patients *know* they are being heard.

D.M.W.

Introduction by Alan B. Ettinger, M.D.

One day in 1995, I found myself in the waiting room of the intensive care unit, not in my role as a physician but instead as a concerned husband. The same respirators that had been used to support the breathing of my patients with uncontrollable seizures were now sustaining the life of my comatose and paralyzed wife, herself a doctor, who had developed a devastating pulmonary illness.

Suddenly, my role changed from that of health care provider to being a patient's family member, and I felt helpless and bewildered. Although I was accustomed to providing answers to my patients, I now found myself confused and scared, as I tried to organize my thoughts in order to ask the right kinds of questions and make the best decisions for my wife under the most adverse of conditions. In what was a previously unimaginable switch, I was no longer the doctor who was in charge; instead I was a family member who was anxious, tearful, and in need of emotional support and advice.

Perhaps it is impossible to truly understand the overwhelming feelings that serious illness engenders until one has been personally touched by it. Words used by my patients, such as *fear*, *depression*, and *anxiety*, began to have new meaning for me. Even the anger that doctors occasionally encounter from their patients became more understandable. Although my wife was awake, she was unable to move or speak, and only rarely did anyone try to communicate with her, understand her needs, or explain to her what was happening. Although I was grateful for the superb medical care she received, I felt powerless and exasperated when the staff did not respond immediately to my wife's needs, and I worried about what was happening when I could not be there. I felt guilty when I had to leave her to attend to our children, as though I were abandoning her.

With few exceptions, I was also disturbed to find that most of the compassion expressed to my wife did not come from doctors, but rather from nurses, clergy, technicians, and housekeeping staff. It occurred to me that there must be something terribly wrong with a medical education system that fails to nurture the capacity of physicians to relate emotionally to their patients. I wondered why doctors know all the right questions to ask when looking for the causes of a headache or a low sodium level, yet they are not expected to ask questions to find out how the patient is coping with illness and how illness is affecting the patient's life?

In my professional life as an epilepsy specialist, I had often asked my patients many questions. When did your seizures begin? How do your seizures look? What antiepileptic drugs are you taking? Although I had always considered myself to be a sensitive doctor, I now began to realize the importance of asking a completely different set of questions. How do you feel about having seizures? Are you getting enough support at home? Are you anxious about having seizures? Is there anything that we can do to help you cope with a difficult situation?

Yet, how could the realities of current medical practice, which involve the necessity of seeing more and more patients in shorter and shorter amounts of time, maintaining voluminous documentation, and many other challenges, be reconciled with an idealistic vision of providing patient care? Struggling with this question, we began to set new goals for ourselves and our patients. One goal was to enhance the efficiency of the office visit in order to permit more time to focus on the issues of the most importance to our patients. In order to achieve this, we began to guide our patients in preparing their medical histories and providing prior evaluations before coming to the office, so that time wasted reconstructing medication doses or prior tests with no information in hand could be avoided, and more time would be available to spend on substantive discussions.

Another objective was to ensure that we addressed the issues of highest importance to our patients. To discipline ourselves in this regard, we asked our patients to put in writing the issues they wanted to talk to the doctor about. Having these notations in the medical record ensures that we will discuss these concerns with our patients.

Another goal was to ensure that we attended to the psychological needs of our patients. In the forms we provided to patients before coming to the office, we asked them to answer questions about a wide range of psychosocial aspects of their lives, and a review of their answers became a standard part of our medical evaluation.

Finally, we sought to empower our patients with knowledge and understanding of the medical evaluation process in order to promote a true partnership between doctor and patient. This book represents the culmination of all of our efforts. Our intention is to demystify the complexities of a visit to the doctor, possible hospitalization, and what a medical evaluation entails.

Very slowly, but quite miraculously, my wife's illness began to recede. She regained consciousness, her paralysis resolved, and the chest tubes were removed. Now she is in good health, and we are blessed with this opportunity to share some of the insights about what we learned from this frightening experience. We hope this book will help others who are confronting the challenges of dealing with difficult medical problems.

How to Use This Book

Although there are numerous health books available, *The Essential Patient Handbook* is a different kind of medical guide. It emphasizes the necessity of understanding the reasoning behind each step of the medical evaluation and can help you prepare your medical history based on your specific symptoms. The easy-to-understand clinical case examples given throughout the book will help you gain insight into the medical evaluation process. Ironically, with on-going medical challenges facing our family, we have had the opportunity to field-test this book and have found it to be an invaluable reference that can be consulted before each doctor visit. We hope you will find it as useful as we do.

> *The Handbook* includes many forms that can be used to prepare a detailed medical history and other information to share with your doctors, in addition to questions you can ask. These forms can be downloaded from the publisher's Web site: www.demosmedpub.com, filled out, and printed on a home computer.

Part I of this book encourages you to take charge of your health care by preparing your medical history before you see the doctor! In doing so, you will learn about the pieces of the puzzle that comprise the medical evaluation, including summarizing the main reason for seeing the doctor, details about your symptoms, prior illnesses, your family's medical history, prior test results, your health habits, how illness affects your quality of life, and ensuring that your doctor has not missed any important details.

Preparation of your medical history takes time and effort. Rather than completing these forms in haste—for example, during an unexpected medical crisis—we advise working on the forms before an acute event occurs, so that background information can be composed in a thoughtful, thorough fashion. Sitting with family members while preparing these forms may help you recall important dates and medical problems. These forms will help you deal with urgent medical situations, but they should also be used to develop a long-term medical record that you can refer to each time you visit a doctor.

Part II deals with special evaluations, including preparing information for the pediatrician, seeing a psychiatrist, providing a history for intellectually-challenged individuals, and preparing advance directives. Be aware, however, that a detailed review of the information you have prepared using this book may not necessarily be appropriate for every office visit. You and your doctor can review this information selectively as it pertains to the issues of your specific medical condition.

Part III will help you prepare the essential questions you need to ask your doctor about diagnosis and treatment. Review these questions before going to the doctor's office. You can also take *The Handbook* with you to the doctor's office so that you will be prepared to ask the important questions.

While many doctors welcome the opportunity to work with well-informed patients, be aware that some health care providers may be resistant and sometimes even hostile to people who ask too many questions. We find this attitude unacceptable. Issues surrounding this reaction by doctors and suggestions for dealing with this problem are highlighted in Chapter 17: "The Good, the Bad and the Ugly—Do Not Let Difficult Doctors Get on Your Case."

Part IV concludes with a variety of topics that will also assist you in handling doctor-patient interactions, such as the preparation of billing information, educating yourself before seeing the doctor, analyzing the diverse types of feelings you may experience in different medical situations, and surviving a hospital stay.

But what if you think you have a good doctor who takes the time to ask you a lot of questions and listens to your responses? You may say, "Why do I need to prepare all this information?" Remember, no matter how great your doctor is *you* know your symptoms and your body the best. Even a great doctor can use your help in collecting and organizing the information that will lead to the most accurate diagnosis and the best treatment.

Our book emphasizes the need for optimum communication with your physician. In our opinion, the failure of a doctor to provide reasonable time for discussion with a patient represents a major deficiency in health care delivery and should not be viewed as an acceptable norm in today's health care. Our hope is that this book may contribute to the establishment of empathetic communication during the medical interview as a standard and integral part of any medical evaluation. We look forward to the day when talking to a patient about the complexities of a medical problem and its treatment will be as essential as taking a blood pressure or tapping a reflex.

PART I

The Medical Evaluation Process & Developing Your Own Medical Record

CHAPTER 1

What Are You Complaining About? – The Chief Complaint

Imagine that you are the manager of an auto repair shop. One morning, Mr. Jones brings in his car for repair. He meets you at the desk and reports, "I woke up this morning, looked out the window, and noticed it was raining. I had breakfast and then got ready for work. Then I got into my car and turned on the windshield wipers. I decided to take the highway. I drove for about three miles at 45 mph and then decided to turn on the radio. Later, I had to slow down because there was a large patch of ice on the road. I started out on Route 45 and then got off at the 2nd exit, going east...."

You might continue to listen patiently, collecting the details of the story, and waiting to hear how this led to an automobile repair issue. Alternatively, you may decide to interrupt Mr. Jones and inquire, "Before you go into further detail, what is the main reason you are bringing your car in for repair?"

Mr. Jones might respond, "I heard a new rattling sound coming from the back of the car," and then proceed to give you more details while you make specific inquiries about the problems with his car.

What is the advantage of getting to the main idea first rather than listening to the entire story as originally presented? One reason is that it is difficult to remember the details of a story without having a specific target question or goal in mind. Understanding the punch line of a story in the beginning allows the listener to understand what elements of the story are needed to clarify the problem and which features are less important to remember. While none of us would describe our automobile troubles in the way that Mr. Jones did, it is not uncommon for patients to present their medical problems to their doctor in this fashion. A better alternative to the approach taken by Mr. Jones would be to express the primary reason for seeking medical attention at the beginning of the interview. Further details can be stated later. The main problem or specific reason for a medical visit is referred to by doctors as the *chief complaint*. Clarifying the chief complaint at the beginning of the interview gives a focus to the subsequent discussion.

Do not let your doctor drown in details – you may need him someday.

Many people seeking medical care immediately plunge into the details of their medical history. Doctors appreciate receiving as much information as possible, but inundating your doctor all at once can actually make it difficult for him to take an organized history. Once the chief complaint is identified, the doctor has a goal or target symptom to focus on and can then integrate or dismiss the information you give him selectively, as they pertain to the problem. If the chief complaint has not been identified, however, your doctor will struggle to retain every detail and will be unsure if each one is important in clarifying an undisclosed main problem. You will have plenty of opportunity to go into detail when you prepare your *History of Present Illness* (HPI), discussed in the next chapter.

Sometimes it is difficult to formulate a specific complaint. For example, you may say, "I'm here because I'm supposed to see a doctor again." A more useful communication would be, "I have suffered from high blood pressure for 10 years, and I am here to have my blood pressure checked and receive my annual physical." This is the type of communication we encourage for specific complaints.

Do not play doctor when you explain your chief complaint.

If you answer your doctor's question, "What brings you to the office or hospital?" with "I came in a taxi with my Uncle Vinnie," you are being a little too literal in your response. Similarly, telling the doctor your opinion as to the diagnosis rather than stating specific symptoms is not the best response either. For example, if you have *diabetes mellitus* and have experienced new dizziness you could tell the doctor you want to be seen because your diabetes is not being sufficiently controlled. However, a better answer would be, "I have starting having dizzy spells." Later on, tell your doctor you suspect that lack of control of your diabetes is the cause. You do not want to encourage your doctor to think in narrow terms rather than consider the broad range of diagnostic possibilities.

What if there are many reasons for seeing the doctor?

When you have difficulty narrowing your symptoms down to one problem, rather than simply writing down one symptom on the chief complaint form, you can prepare a list of the main problems and indicate how long each has been going on.

For example:

- Headache for one year, worse over the past two weeks
- Palpitations for three months
- Swelling of the left leg for the past two weeks

With this list in hand, you and your doctor can determine which symptoms should take priority. The doctor will prioritize by making brief general inquiries into each area. You and your doctor may also choose to postpone discussing the details of one or more symptoms until a subsequent office visit, in order to allow a more thorough discussion of the most pressing symptom.

The "Oh, did I mention..." syndrome.

Perhaps you have not read about this in the newspapers this year but, in fact, there is an epidemic of this syndrome in doctors' offices across the country. Even Mr. Jones was afflicted with it.

After dropping off his car at the repair shop, Mr. Jones told the doctor he was concerned about a minor rash on his left arm. After a history, examination, and a reassuring discussion with the doctor about the rash, Mr. Jones was about to leave when he happened to mention, "Oh, by the way; last night I developed an excruciating headache, the worst of my life, and it still hurts."

Although the doctor has just spent half an hour looking at a relatively inconsequential rash, he is now sweating bullets about possible internal bleeding in Mr. Jones' head. The doctor has to start the interview all over again. Had he known earlier on about the headache, he would undoubtedly have directed his primary attention to that problem first.

Sometimes the symptoms that are mentioned at the end of a visit relate to more sensitive subjects, such as sexual issues, psychosocial problems, or psychological difficulties. Identifying these issues earlier in the interview will make sure that these very important topics are discussed (see further discussion in Chapter 8).

Why now?

Your chief complaint does not have to be a symptom that started recently. Perhaps it has been occurring for a long period of time but you have only recently become concerned because the symptom has worsened or has become intolerable. Maybe a report on television or a frightening story you heard from a friend about similar symptoms has heightened your worries about your own problems. Perhaps you are convinced that the symptom means you are going to die or that it will prevent you from getting around each day. Are you getting depressed about it? Tell your doctor what your worst fears are about your medical symptoms. It is well worth it; your doctor may be able to offer reassurance or clarify any misconceptions that you may have. Sometimes, the specific symptom may not be as important as the opportunity to meet with your doctor and discuss other more sensitive topics or concerns. A good doctor should delve deeper into all aspects of the chief complaint and help you identify the issues of greatest importance to you.

Your chief complaint is not necessarily the same as your most severe medical problem. For example, the doctor may want to talk with you about your back pain, but you may be more concerned about having headaches. The issues you decide to raise with the doctor also reveal valuable information about how you feel your symptoms affect your quality of life and activities of daily living. For example, your friend may not mind feeling sleepy from a medication, but for you this may be devastating in that it interferes with your ability to function. Some symptoms may be embarrassing or difficult to discuss openly. A good doctor engages in a sensitive discussion of symptoms and the strong feelings they evoke. Your selection of what symptoms to emphasize helps the doctor focus on those symptoms and on the context in which they appear. If you feel that the doctor is not focusing on the problem that concerns you the most, let the doctor know.

Now that you have prepared your chief complaint you are ready to prepare the details about your medical problem. The next chapter will explain the best way to do that.

FORM 1

Chief Complaint

In a few words, list the reason or reasons you are being evaluated by the doctor, including both the problem(s) and how long each has occurred.

_____

_____

_____

_____

_____

_____

_____

_____

_____

_____

_____

_____

CHAPTER 2

Make Your Mark in History— Your History of Present Illness

"In a matter of weeks, however, my vision worsened so rapidly I had to consult an ophthalmologist. He prescribed reading glasses, which helped considerably for a while. But when we began filming, I started to experience other strange things that concerned me. Every now and then I would feel a cold tingling sensation in my feet that would come and go for no apparent reason. Once we started shooting out on the beach, I found it difficult to keep my balance in the sand. Several times the simple act of getting up from a sitting position left me feeling wildly off kilter, as if I'd been spinning. It is hard to explain, but for a few seconds I would feel as if I had no sense of balance at all. Frankie, noticing something was not right, helped me up, then joked, 'Annette, I think you've had a little too much to drink!'"

ANNETTE FUNICELLO
A Dream is a Wish Your Heart Makes: My Story

What's the story?

The story of your symptoms, such as that described above by Annette Funicello long before she was diagnosed with multiple sclerosis, is very important. Now that your doctor has an understanding of your chief complaint, it is time to tell the story about your symptoms in detail. Effective storytellers know that a story needs to be organized and that it should include information describing the setting, when the story takes place, who the characters are, and what happened. The story about your symptoms that you tell to your doctor also needs to be very organized. The name of this story is the *History of Present Illness* (HPI). The HPI is important whenever you develop new symptoms that need to be described to the doctor. The HPI may be the single most important part of your entire medical evaluation. Despite all the new fancy MRIs and nuclear scans you hear about on the news each day, there is nothing more valuable in arriving at a diagnosis than a doctor and patient spending the time to get a complete history.

Entering information into your HPI is very different than mindlessly punching numbers into a calculator and waiting for the final tally. Rather than asking a series of random questions and then analyzing the answers at the end, a good doctor will carefully select each question and decide on the next question based on the earlier answers. The questions your doctor asks in the HPI are each linked to possible diagnoses that can explain your symptoms. Each diagnosis has its own typical characteristics, including how the associated symptoms begin, how long they last, and how they usually feel. Even with as little to go on as the chief complaint, an experienced doctor can select the relevant questions, the answers to which either support or go against each possible diagnosis.

How the doctor decides what questions to ask.

When your doctor hears your answer to a question, he selects his next question based on your preceding answer. For example, perhaps you see your doctor for a cough and he asks you whether the cough is dry or productive of *sputum* (phlegm). If the answer is productive, she may probe further by asking about the nature of the sputum—for example, whether it contains blood, what color it is, and how much is produced.

I am trying to give my doctor as much information as possible, but he keeps interrupting me with questions!

Sometimes people feel insulted because when they answer a doctor's question, the doctor immediately moves on to another subject without listening for further details. Assuming that your doctor is not distracted because he is thinking about his upcoming vacation to Florida, a more likely explanation is that he has a lot of ground to cover in a relatively short amount of time. When answers to questions do not clarify a possible diagnosis, the doctor may shift to other questions, fishing for clues that explain the symptom. The doctor usually focuses on the details after getting an idea about what the diagnosis may be.

How can I prepare answers to questions I have not heard yet?

How can you possibly prepare your answers if you have not heard the questions because you have not met the doctor yet? Despite the wide diversity of questions that could be potentially asked during a clinical interview, there tends to be a stereotypical list of questions that are asked, irrespective of specific symptoms. Just think about the last time you saw a doctor for pain in your stomach, a headache, weakness, numbness, or some other symptom. Your doctor probably asked questions such as:

- When did the symptom start?
- What makes it worse?

- What makes it better?
- How does it feel?
- How long did it last?

Some of these questions may take a little thought before you can answer. Therefore, it would be best to think about your answers to potential questions *before* you see the doctor. That way you can take your time preparing your answers; you might even ask a friend or family member for help in recalling the details. The two HPI forms including in this book each have a complete list of typical questions that you can review before you visit your doctor. Keeping such a record can also be helpful for recalling details at a later time, such as when you see another doctor.

Form 2A can be used when you experience symptoms that have occurred more than once—for example, recurrent abdominal pain or headaches. It is especially useful to describe the history of recurring symptoms associated with a chronic illness. Form 2B is appropriate for a one-time event that has either persisted or gone away.

HOW TO ANSWER THE QUESTIONS

Timing Of Symptoms:

At what age or date did the episodes begin?

Do not worry if you cannot recall the exact date that a problem started. A good estimate usually suffices. On the other hand, try to avoid vague terms, such as *recently*, which for some people means a week ago and for others it means three months ago. For example, when the author of this book, Alan Ettinger, tells his wife Deborah Weisbrot that he cleaned up the garage recently, he really means three years ago.

Keep a calendar and mark down when episodes occurred for easy reference. Other questions related to timing of symptoms may include:

At what age or date did the episodes stop (if applicable)?

What is the average frequency of episodes in a given day, month, or year?

What is the maximum number of episodes you have experienced in a given day, month, or year?

Precipitating And Modifying Factors:

Is there anything, such as lack of sleep or drinking alcohol, that tends to bring on the episodes?

This is important. For example, if you experience abdominal pain every time you eat fatty French fries at the local fast-food joint, this may be a clue to gall bladder disease, among other possibilities.

Were there any changes in your medications, such as starting a new medication or reducing a medication, when the episodes began?

One of the most common mistakes in medical care is to forget about the effects of medication. Also, do not neglect mentioning non-prescription medicines, herbs, and other supplements.

Is there anything that makes an episode worse once it has begun?

It is not just the old joke: "Doctor, when I do this, it hurts," and the doctor answers, "So don't do it." This type of inquiry actually gives a clue about the cause of the problem.

What do you typically do in response to having an episode?

Certain reactions in response to certain symptoms may also point to a specific kind of diagnosis.

Is there anything that tends to give you relief?

For example, Joe suffers from recurrent headaches. Each time he has a headache, he retreats to a dark room, withdrawing from bright lights and loud sounds. This is a classic response to symptoms of a migraine headache.

Is there anything you have tried to do to make yourself feel better that did not work?

Even though the doctor is mostly concerned about making the diagnosis, it does not hurt to start thinking ahead about treatments that may be offered. If something did not work in the past, maybe it is worth trying something else. Also, a good or bad response to a treatment can give more clues about the diagnosis.

Circumstances:

These questions provide a setting for the symptoms:

What are you typically doing when symptoms begin?
Are there any warning signs that an episode is going to occur?
Do episodes tend to occur at any particular place?
Do episodes tend to occur at any particular time?

Description:

Do you have any associated symptoms before, during, or after an episode?

The context in which symptoms occur and the company they keep helps the doctor narrow down the wide differential diagnosis.

List your experiences during an episode from start to finish, step-by-step.

This is an opportunity to describe what has occurred in detail and to organize it in a logical fashion that everyone can understand.

List what others observe when you have an episode from start to finish, step-by-step.

It is amazing how your own experience can differ from what someone else observed. Combining all accounts yields a wealth of information for the doctor.

How long does an episode last?

What symptoms do you experience after an episode is over?

Sometimes, there is a distinct period after symptoms are gone during which new symptoms appear.

Answer the following questions if they apply to you:

Where is the symptom located?

Be as specific as possible. If the symptom involves a small area, point to that spot. If the symptom radiates from one region to another, mention all the areas involved.

How does the symptom feel?

This question describes what is called the *quality* of the symptom. Try to describe the symptom with regard to timing. For example, is it constant or does it come and go? Is it continuous, but then it gets slightly worse or better over time?

Use descriptive terms, such as *sharp, dull, stabbing, pounding*, or *steady*. Here is an analogy. Which statement conveys more about the feeling you had when you got the doctor's bill? (1) I was upset, or (2) I was frustrated, enraged, and I had a severe, pounding pain in the back of my head?

How severe is the symptom? (Rate from 1 to 10; one is least and 10 is worst.)

In addition to rating the severity, consider using descriptive terms, such as "mild enough for me to ignore it most of the time," "so severe, I could not concentrate on anything I was doing," or "the worst pain I have ever experienced."

Are the symptoms getting worse or better in severity or frequency?

Your doctor better know about it if your symptoms are getting worse! This could be a red flag that something needs to be done pronto!

Effect On Function:

The next few questions speak to the importance of not only the symptom, but the potentially profound affect the symptom may have on all of the facets of one's life. These questions include:

How do the symptoms affect your functioning?

Are you disabled by the symptoms?

How do symptoms affect your mood?

How do symptoms affect your relationships, occupation, and home life?

These kinds of questions are less crucial for diagnosis but are more important for understanding how the problem affects your quality of life. While the medical profession is often accused of being insensitive to the effects of illness on the person, these questions ensure that these important aspects receive a prominent role in the discussion with your doctor.

Cause Of Symptoms And Possible Fears About Them:

New symptoms often provoke tremendous fear about dreadful diagnoses, such as cancer. These feelings are often not shared with the doctor. This is unfortunate, since in many cases the doctor can clarify misconceptions and offer reassurance. These questions include:

Have you ever received a diagnosis for these symptoms?

What are your ideas about what may be causing the symptoms?

What is your worst fear about what is causing the symptoms and the problems they create?

Miscellaneous Questions:

Have you had similar episodes in the past?

Sometimes, the interview is so focused on the present symptoms that your doctor forgets to ask if you ever had the problem before. If you did, that could change everything.

Have you witnessed or been directly exposed to anyone around you who has had similar symptoms?

This can be a clue to potentially contagious, toxic, or genetically-determined causes. Even psychologically-driven symptoms are modeled after symptoms that someone else experienced.

What if there is more than one chief complaint?

If the problems are important to you, you need to spend the time answering questions about each problem separately. Remember, however, that it may not be feasible to cover all areas of concern in one visit to your doctor. In this situation, you and your doctor should decide which issues should be discussed now and which can be deferred to a later visit.

Here are two examples of why it makes sense to prepare your HPI ahead of time:

> Mr. Harris is a 32-year-old man who is being evaluated for seizures, which can be understood as electrical "storms" in the brain. When asked how often the seizures occur, he vaguely replies, "a lot." The doctor asks "Once a day? Once a month? Once a year?" Mr. Harris replies, "I think a few times per year." When asked what happens during a seizure, Mr. Harris responds, "I don't know; I'm not conscious when they happen and I don't remember them." He is also unsure when the seizures began. Ultimately Mr. Harris exclaims, "Why are you asking me so many questions? You're the doctor; you're the one who should know the answers."

> Mr. Kaufman, on the other hand, is a 50-year-old man who is being evaluated for episodes of dizziness. He has prepared detailed information about the dizzy spells, including their frequency of four times per year, their onset at age 48, their spinning quality, associated ringing sounds in his right ear, his diminished hearing in that ear, and the absence of prior medical risk factors, such as ear infections or medication intake.

To answer the question asked by Mr. Harris: yes, the doctor should ultimately provide some answers, but how can that be done without even the most fundamental information? Mr. Harris did not invest any effort to help his doctor figure out the problem, and he was completely passive, depending on the doctor to figure everything out. Mr. Kaufman, on the other hand, has thoughtfully prepared the kind of information that is likely to be asked during a clinical interview and, therefore, he does not need to spend much time reflecting on each question asked by the doctor. Even before performing the examination, the doctor has already thought of many possible diagnoses, such as a disorder of the balance centers of the ear and, much less likely, a neurologic problem. Giving and receiving detailed information efficiently has another benefit: it leaves more time at the end of the visit for the doctor to discuss the diagnosis and explain in more detail how it should be treated.

The next chapter will help you prepare for questions that are specific to your particular medical symptom if your symptoms fall into one of the more common types.

FORM 2A

History of Present Illness
Recurrent Episodes

Timing of Symptoms:

At what age or on what date did the episodes begin? _____

At what age or on what date did the episodes stop? (If applicable.) _____

What is the average frequency of episodes in a given day, month or year?____

_____

What is the maximum number of episodes you have experienced in a given day, month, or year? _____

Circumstances:

What are you typically doing when it comes on? _____

_____

Are there any warning feelings that an episode is going to occur? _____

_____

Is there any particular place you are at when the episode occurs?_____

_____

Is there any particular time when the episode occurs? _____

Description:

Do you have any associated symptoms around the time or during an episode? _____

_____

List what you experience during an episode step-by-step, from start to finish:_____

_____

List what others have observed when you have an episode step-by-step, from start to finish: _____

_____

_____

How long does an episode last? _____

What symptoms do you experience after an episode is over? _____

_____

Where is the symptom located? (If applicable.) _____

How does the symptom feel? (This question describes what is known as the *quality* of the symptom. Use descriptive terms, such as *sharp, dull, stabbing, pounding,* and *steady,* to explain the symptom. Also note if the symptom is steady, intermittent versus continuous, or unchanged versus waxing and waning. _____

_____

_____

How severe is the symptom? (Rate from 1-10; one is least and 10 is worst.) In addition to rating the severity, use descriptive terms. _____

_____

Are the symptoms getting worse or better in severity or frequency? _____

Precipitants and Modifying Factors:

Is there anything, such as lack of sleep or drinking alcohol, that tends to bring on the episodes? _____

Were there any changes in your medications, such as starting a new medication or reducing a medication, when the episodes began? _____

Is there anything that makes an episode worse once it has begun? _____

What do you typically do in response to having an episode? _____

_____

Is there anything that tends to give you relief? _____

_____

Is there anything you have tried to do to make yourself feel better that did NOT work? _____

_____

Effect on Function:

How do the symptoms affect your functioning? _____

_____

Are you disabled by the symptoms? _____

How do symptoms affect your mood? _____

_____

How do symptoms affect your relationships, occupation, and home life? ____

_____

Cause of Symptoms and Possible Fears About Them:

Have you ever received a diagnosis for these symptoms? _____

_____

What are your ideas about what may be causing the symptoms? _____

_____

What is your worst fear about what is causing the symptoms, or about the problems they may create for you? _____

_____

Miscellaneous:

Have you had similar episodes in the past? _____

_____

Have you witnessed or been directly exposed to anyone around you who has had similar symptoms? _____

_____

History of Present Illness
Single Event

Timing and Circumstances:

Where were you when it came on? _____

What were you doing when it came on? _____

When did it begin? _____

Were there any warning feelings that an episode was about to occur? _____

_____

Did the symptoms stop? If so, when? How long did the symptoms last? ____

_____

Description:

List what you experienced step-by-step, from start to finish. _____

_____

List what others observed step-by-step, from start to finish. _____

_____

If the symptoms stopped, what did you experience afterwards? _____

_____

Where is (was) the symptom located? (If applicable.) _____

How does (did) the symptom feel? _____

_____

How severe is (was) the symptom? (Rate from 1-10; one is least and 10 is
worst.) _____

Are the symptoms getting worse, better, or have they stopped? _____

_____

Specify any associated symptoms. _____

_____

Precipitants and Modifying Factors:

Is there anything that brings on the symptoms, such as lack of sleep or
drinking alcohol? _____

Was there any change in your medications, such as starting a medication or reducing a medication, when the episode began? _____

Once the symptoms began, did anything make it worse? _____

_____

What did you do in response to having the symptoms? _____

_____

Did anything tend to make the symptoms better? _____

_____

Did anything you tried to make it better *not* work? _____

_____

Effect on Function:

How did the symptoms affect your functioning? _____

Were you disabled by the symptoms? _____

How did the symptom affect your mood? _____

If this is a longstanding problem, how did the symptoms affect your relationships, occupation, or home life? _____

Cause of Symptoms and Possible Fears About Them:

Did you receive a diagnosis for these symptoms? _____

What are your ideas about what may be causing the symptoms? _____

_____

What is your worst fear about what is causing the symptoms and the problems they create? _____

_____

Miscellaneous:

Have you had similar episodes in the past? _____

Did you witness, or have you been directly exposed to, anyone who has had similar symptoms? _____

CHAPTER 3

Your Specific Symptoms[1]

> "When you finish reading a murder mystery, all the clues that led to the discovery of the culprit seem obvious, although they were often not at all apparent at the time. So, too, when a patient's illness has resolved, either in a cure or in death, the major facts of his disease seem obvious in retrospect. The clues that should have been explored immediately, chest X-rays or slightly abnormal lab values, the tests that should have been done, all seem abundantly clear, though at the time the doctor is working through a series of educated guesses, sifting through facts and theories, to find an answer. Each illness starts out as a mystery, and so it is inevitable that mistakes will be made as the mystery is solved. The wrong person is accused – it is the liver! – and then it turns out to be the lungs. The bullets from the suspected murder weapon do not match the bullets in the victim; the organism in the laboratory is not the one suspected and though they may appear to be errors when the case is closed, the mysterious nature of disease means that some of them are inevitable and must be forgiven – hard as it is to accept this fact when the effects of the illness are felt on the body."

JAMIE WEISMAN
As I Live and Breathe

While the preceding chapter provided general questions applicable to most kinds of symptoms, this chapter provides supplementary questions applicable to specific symptoms. This list includes some of the most common symptoms encountered by the general practitioner. Refer to the relevant section of this chapter if you suffer from any of the following:

- Amenorrhea
- Bleeding from the rectum
- Confusion or memory difficulties
- Cough
- Dizziness or vertigo
- Fatigue
- Fever
- Gastrointestinal symptoms (constipation or diarrhea)

1. Adapted in part from: *The Complete Patient History* by M. Kraytman. New York: McGraw-Hill Book Company, 1979.

- High blood pressure
- Insomnia
- Loss of consciousness, fainting, or seizures
- Nausea or vomiting
- Pain in the abdomen (belly)
- Pain in the chest
- Pain or swelling in a joint
- Pain in the head or face
- Pain in the neck or upper or lower back
- Palpitations (fluttering in the chest)
- Shortness of breath
- Sleepiness
- Swelling
- Frequent urination
- Weakness
- Weight loss (with or without loss of appetite)

Responses to these questions can be prepared before visiting the doctor and will further enhance the quality of the medical interview.

Amenorrhea

Amenorrhea refers to missing the normally expected menstrual period for a significant amount of time. Information to prepare for the doctor should include the date of your last period, how many periods were missed, previous menstrual history, including age that menstruation began and typical degree of regularity, symptoms suggesting possible current pregnancy, current stress, whether it began after a gynecological procedure or delivery, and associated symptoms, such as headache, visual changes, depression, nausea and vomiting, increased hair growth throughout the body, loss of hair in the armpit and groin areas, change in skin coloring, vaginal bleeding, milk secretion from the breasts, recent difficulty tolerating cold or hot temperatures in the environment, new marks on the skin, weakness, fever, cough, change in weight, hot flashes, or night sweats. Also describe the nature of your diet and exercise program, and any prior history of gynecological or brain surgeries.

Bleeding From the Rectum

Prepare information for your doctor about the extent of the bleeding. For example, were there streaks of blood or more substantial bleeding, was the bleeding only on the toilet paper or surface of stools, or was it in the toilet water and/or mixed in with stool. Associated symptoms should also be described, including severe fatigue after the blood was noticed, vomiting, change in recent bowel habits, diarrhea, abdominal pain, pain around the anal region, fever, pain on having a bowel movement, bleeding associated with straining at having a bowel movement, bleeding from other parts of the body, and recent and prior travel history. Specify any prior established gastrointestinal diagnoses.

Confusion or Memory Difficulties

If the symptoms are severe, these questions should be completed by others observing the affected individual. Be specific about the problem. For example, have there been new problems in memory, level of alertness, speech, basic orientation to time and place, knowing names of people in the family, counting change or balancing a checkbook, or in common knowledge, such as names or people in the news, recent presidents or important dates in history? Citing specific examples of problems in any of these areas gives more meaning to the description.

Prepare answers to questions that relate to potential causes of change in mental functioning, including respiratory problems, infectious illnesses, such as *meningitis* or *encephalitis* (inflammation of fluid around the brain or the brain itself), tick bites, history of traveling outside the area, known brain abnormalities, heart disease, recent vaccinations, autoimmune disease such as lupus, blood clotting abnormalities, new medications used, recent exposure or withdrawal from alcohol or drugs, exposure to chemicals or toxins at home or in the workplace, known kidney or liver disease, known metabolic problems, such as low sodium in the bloodstream, malnutrition, eating unusual foods, such as herbs or excess vitamins, known sleep problems, exhaustion, or underlying psychiatric disorder.

Cough

In describing the nature of the cough, the doctor will be interested to learn whether the cough is dry or produces sputum (phlegm). Even before submitting a sputum specimen to a laboratory for analysis, a description of the sputum can be highly diagnostic, especially for various types of infection. Therefore, the doctor will want to know the color of the sputum, whether it contains blood, and whether it has a particular odor. Accompanying symptoms, such as pain, fever, shortness of breath, chest pain or weight loss, should be conveyed. Modifying factors that bring it on, such as smoking, taking medicine, or changing posture, as well as maneuvers which improve the cough, can be very helpful to know. Occupational exposure to toxins or fumes should be mentioned.

Dizziness or Vertigo

Dizziness means different things for different people and, therefore, trying to match symptoms to descriptions the following can be helpful—for example, sensation of motion or frank spinning, motion sickness, lightheadedness, floating feelings, feeling giddy, feeling as if you have left your body, fogginess, cloudiness, or feeling off-balance.

If dizziness refers to a sense of motion or spinning, specify further whether you felt yourself moving or had the sensation that the world around you was moving and in which direction. You should also indicate what precipitates or worsens the dizzy feeling, such as any particular position of the head or body, or from taking a medication. Associated symptoms, such as ringing, roaring, or fullness feelings in the ear, nausea, vomiting, weakness in facial or limb muscles, sensation abnormalities, headache, or hearing loss, should be outlined.

Fatigue

Fatigue refers to an overwhelming feeling of lack of energy. Be prepared to describe what times of the day you experience fatigue, how physical or mental effort is related to the fatigue, and whether rest or sleep relieves the fatigue. Questions about home life, work, relationships stresses, and mood are particularly important for the doctor to know. The doctor will also want to know about the nature of your daily diet, current medications, and associated symptoms of possible illness, such as fever, cough, night sweats, weight gain or loss, appetite changes, sleep problems, or weakness of a specific part of the body. Details about past medical history, including recent infections, heart condition, and alcohol problems, should be conveyed to the doctor.

Fever

Fever is formally defined as a sign that can be measured rather than a symptom. When fever occurs in the absence of an obvious cause, the doctor will cast a wide net of questions looking for symptoms referable to a specific body part. Therefore, include any new symptoms, such as excessive sweating, night sweats, chest discomfort, cough (including coughing up phlegm), shortness of breath, headaches, earaches, toothache, joint pains, muscle pains, back pains, sore throat, hoarseness, change in urination or bowel habits, nausea and vomiting, red eyes, stiff neck, rash, swollen glands, any recent new medications, and recent exposures to people with illnesses. The doctor may also ask you about recent and prior travel history, the work you do, exposure to birds or other wild animals, your diet, illegal drug use, skin wounds, and prior history of heart valve disease or surgeries.

Gastrointestinal Symptoms (Constipation and Diarrhea)

In order to understand the significance of a change in the frequency or nature of bowel movements, it is helpful to know what bowel function was like before the onset of the symptoms. You should describe characteristics of the stool, including how loose or firm it is, its color, and whether it is accompanied by blood, mucus, or undigested food. Include information as to how the symptoms relate to life stresses, degree of physical inactivity, and diet—for example, the amount of roughage in the diet or recent dietary changes. Tell the doctor about current medications and the use of laxatives. Also include associated symptoms, such as feeling bloated, nausea, vomiting, or abdominal pain.

High Blood Pressure

High blood pressure (hypertension) is a condition, not an actual symptom. In fact, high blood pressure often goes unnoticed until it causes possible complications. Relevant questions include inquiries into how closely the blood pressure has been monitored, how it was detected, what the typical and maximum blood pressure readings have been, and symptoms that may be associated with high blood pressure complications, including shortness of breath, chest pain, headaches, visual problems, and dizziness. Questions related to potential causes of high blood pressure may delve into possible complaints about episodes of sweating with fluttering in the chest and nervousness, and urinary symptoms.

Insomnia

Insomnia usually refers to difficulty falling asleep, and the sleep that is achieved does not feel deep, sufficient, or refreshing. Questions to think about include how many hours do you typically sleep each night, and is there difficulty falling and/or staying asleep?

Describe the nature and amount of your physical and mental activity during a typical day, the amount of caffeine-containing drinks ingested and the time of day you drink them, current medications, medical symptoms that interfere with sleep, how many and how long are the naps you take during the day, abnormal restless sensations in the legs before going to sleep, new problems tolerating heat in the environment with increased sweating or palpitations, anxious or depressed feelings, and any prior psychiatric difficulties. Also note whether your bedmate snores or moves around constantly while you are trying to sleep.

Loss of Consciousness, Fainting, or Seizures

It is very important to get a description about what happened both from the affected individual and from a witness, since the accounts usually differ greatly and both descriptions add much to the understanding of what happened. Many questions listed above in the section about dizziness also apply here. Indicate whether episodes are precipitated by acute bleeding anywhere, excessive heat exposure, drinking alcohol or using drugs, head injury, taking a water pill, eating poorly that day, changes in blood pressure or diabetes medication, experiencing sudden pain or fear from an unpleasant sight, wearing a tight-fitting collar, straining during urination or a bowel movement, extreme coughing, or during hyperventilation (rapid breathing in and out) due to anxiety. Associated symptoms should be noted, such as jerking movements of arms and legs, chest pain, pains in other parts of the body, sweating, change in color in the face or body, shortness of breath, fluttering in the chest, racing heartbeat, tingling around mouth or fingers, headache, shaking of body parts, spinning sensations, anxiety, falling sleep, tongue biting, having loss of urine or stool, muscle soreness, staring, or fixed movements of the eyes.

Nausea and Vomiting

Characteristics of vomiting provide important clues as to the causes of the problem. Vomiting should be described in terms of its frequency, how forceful it is, how sudden or unexpected it occurs, and what symptoms occur along with it—for example, abdominal pain. Be prepared for graphic questions, such as how the vomitus smelled and tasted, and what it appeared to contain—for example, undigested food or blood.

All foods (especially new foods), and alcohol and drug intake over the preceding week should be mentioned. Association of vomiting with a very stressful or anxiety-inducing situation should be noted, if relevant. Describe any other associated symptoms, such as headaches.

Pain in the Abdomen (Belly)

This is one of the most commonly experienced symptoms. One of the important questions concerns the specific location of the pain. Is it in a specific location or is it more generalized? If it is well-localized, be prepared to point to that area for the doctor. Does the pain remain in the same place? Describe the specific timing as to how the pain moves around and changes in intensity. Does the pain travel to the shoulder, the back, the jaw, or into the groin?

Describing the quality and characteristics of pain can also be very revealing about its cause. Is it burning, bloating, achey, cramp-like, crushing, continuous or coming and going, steady or throbbing? Is the pain brought on, worsened, or relieved with any specific body position or any specific food, such as fatty foods or medicines? Is it brought on by being very nervous? Does taking a deep breath or cough worsen the pain? Did you experience nausea and vomiting, belching, constipation (specify when your last bowel movement occurred), diarrhea, blood in the stool, light-colored stool, weight loss, fever, urinary symptoms, and chest pressure? If applicable, specify the time of last menstrual period and relationship to the pain. Make a list of anyone around you who also got sick in a similar way. Past medical history related to the abdomen is obviously crucial—for example, prior abdominal surgery, ulcers, or kidney stones,

Pain in the Chest

This can be a particularly serious symptom and providing an organized, detailed description is invaluable in helping the doctor find the specific causes. Point to the location of the pain and indicate whether it radiates anywhere— for example, to an arm, neck, shoulder. Describe how it feels. Is there tightness, pressure, or burning? Indicate any associated symptoms, such as fluttering in the chest, rapid heart beat, shortness of breath, cough, nausea, or a cold clammy feeling. Mention any position that worsens the pain, such as leaning forward.

Pain or Swelling in a Joint

Information to prepare includes listing every joint location where pain or swelling is experienced. Indicate whether the symptoms occur in individual, repeating attacks or if they have been persistent, whether the pains migrate from one joint to another, whether joint swelling developed before, after, or during joint pain, whether pains occur at rest, after prolonged inactivity or only with movement (including the type and duration of movement), and whether injury or drinking alcohol preceded the attack. Describe associated symptoms, such as fever, chills, muscle pains, swallowing difficulties, cough, shortness of breath, back pain, eye problems, pain or significant change in color of the skin of the hands in response to cold temperatures, and pain when urinating or penile discharge. Indicate any prior sore throat, vaccinations, prior similar attacks, and any family history of joint problems.

Pain in the Head or Face

Describe any prior history of headaches and how they compare to the current headache. Clarify how rapidly the headache began, the specific location of the pain and any associated symptoms, such as neck pain, tearing in the eye, nasal stuffiness, fever, visual changes, nausea, nose bleeds, confusion, weakness or numbness in a part of the body. Describe how the headaches feel; are they steady, throbbing, pounding, sharp like a knife, pressure, continuous, waxing and waning, dull, or aching? Indicate whether coughing, sneezing, bending over, flexing the neck, or anything else tends to worsen the headache. Include any other possible provoking factors, such as lack of sleep or intake of alcohol or drugs.

Pain in the Neck, or Upper or Lower Back

For these types of symptoms, it is essential to be precise about the location of the pain and where it may travel to—for example, radiating to the inner portion of the thigh or the back side of the hand towards the thumb. Consider drawing a picture of the body and relating exactly where the pain is present. Use descriptive terms, such as *sharp, dull, stabbing*, or *burning*. Factors that precipitated the original pain or worsen the current pain should be noted, including a recent fall or back injury, prolonged sitting, lifting, new physical activity, coughing, sneezing, walking, or recent prolonged use of medications. Body positions that worsen or relieve the pain should be stated—for example, lying flat, lying with knees bent, standing, or leaning forward. Mention any new weakness or numbness in a limb, loss of control over bowel or bladder function, pain or burning on urination, and difficulty feeling the sensation of passing urine or moving the bowels. Men should note any recent problems attaining an erection; women should describe any relationship between pain and the menstrual cycle, or vaginal discharge.

Palpitations

Palpitations are fluttering sensations in the chest or a sensation in the chest of a run of heartbeats. When the heart is beating rapidly due to exercise, the sensation of the heartbeat is normal. Medical conditions, such as thyroid disease, heart disease, anemia, fever, drugs (including appetite suppressants, cold remedies, and caffeine), and drug withdrawal—for example, stopping Valium® abruptly—raise the heart rate significantly and can also cause palpitations. Sometimes, anxiety in the absence of a medical condition can heighten awareness of the heartbeat and be perceived as palpitations.

Even in the absence of a rapid heart rate, irregular heart beats can give rise to the sensation of palpitation. In describing palpitations, you should be very specific about how long the episodes last. If the pulse is taken during an episode, tell the doctor about the heart rate and if it was irregular. Note any associated symptoms, such as fainting feeling, nervousness, sweating, chest pain or pressure, or shortness of breath.

Shortness of Breath

Describe what you mean by shortness of breath. For example, does your breathing feel shallow or full? Is taking a breath limited by pain? Mention associated symptoms, such as stuffy nose, cough, wheezing, and tingling around the mouth or fingers. Indicate whether shortness of breath occurs at rest or is precipitated by exertion. Specify the typical time of year when symptoms occur and whether there has been exposure to pollen or to others who are currently having respiratory illnesses. Note any relation of shortness of breath to times of emotional upset or stress.

Sleepiness

Excess sleepiness is often associated with but is distinct from fatigue, as described above. Questions to think about include how long the problem has been occurring, whether the feeling of needing to sleep is irresistible, what times of the day the urge to sleep occurs, how long you sleep during the day and at night, whether you wake up feeling refreshed from a nap during the day, and is there any associated sudden loss of muscle power brought on by strong emotions. At the onset of sleep, do you experience difficulty moving or speaking; do you see or hear things that are not really there (hallucinations)? Describe other medical problems, such as obesity, headaches, prior problems affecting the brain, and any family history of sleep problems.

Swelling

Swelling (edema) refers to an abnormal increase in fluid into the tissues of the body outside of the blood vessels. The causes of swelling are dependent on whether the swelling involves the general body or specific body parts. Questions to be anticipated include inquiries into the exact location of the swelling, how quickly the swelling developed, if the swelling is worse during any part of the day, or precipitated by any specific foods or emotional stress. It is also worth thinking about whether the swelling gets worse after standing for a very long time and if it is relieved by lifting the legs. Any associated symptoms, such as chest pain, shortness of breath, bowel or bladder symptoms, leg pains, warm red areas on the leg, or fever, should be discussed with the doctor.

Frequent Urination

Important information includes whether the urination problem began suddenly or gradually, impressions about how much urine is actually made each day and how much this varies from day to day, the typical quantity with each time of urination, how many times urination occurs in a day, any associated pain, whether the need to urinate wakes you up and how many times it does per night, and whether urination occurs more frequently at night than during the day. Inform the doctor about your degree of thirst, whether the frequent urination occurs even on days of reduced fluid intake, and any changes in appetite, weight loss, pains, change in vision, prior injuries or surgeries involving the brain, previous psychiatric difficulties, or prior kidney or prostate diagnoses.

Weakness

In its purest definition, *weakness* refers to actual diminished muscle strength and needs to be distinguished from *fatigue*, a more generalized feeling of lack of energy or being tired. If you are experiencing weakness in one or more parts of your body, you should note whether the weakness is constant or fluctuates, exactly where the weakness is experienced, what specific tasks are difficult to perform, including climbing stairs, getting out of a chair, wiggling your fingers, or combing your hair, and whether the symptoms are progressing. The diagnosis of the cause for weakness is often preceded by the company of symptoms that it keeps. Therefore, you should be prepared to tell the doctor about any other accompanying symptoms, such as pain, numbness, change in bowel and bladder function, confusion, or change in speech or vision.

Once the doctor has an idea of where the weakness is coming from anatomically, she may ask more questions in order to exclude a wide variety of different categories of illness, such as problems affecting blood vessels, infections, degenerative disorders, among many other possibilities.

Weight Loss (With or Without Loss of Appetite)

Be prepared to provide information about prior weight measurements, such as average weight, maximum or minimum weight in the past, how many pounds were lost and how long this has been occurring, current eating habits or recent diets, smoking and daily alcohol intake, stresses, abdominal discomfort, constipation, recent poor tolerance of heat with palpitations or sweating, relation to taking specific medications, changes in the frequency of urination, change in bowel habits, nausea or vomiting, fever, other medical symptoms, and recent changes in mood. Mention whether food tastes bad, if there is any throat pain, or if yellow discoloration of skin has occurred.

Now that you have thoroughly explained your symptoms, it is time to provide your doctor with information about your prior medical problems and how they may relate to your current symptoms. This is explained in the next chapter.

CHAPTER 4

Blast From the Past—
Your Past Medical History

If dealing with the medical profession were anything like a TV game show, the question might sound like this:

> Now, Mr. Smith, we've come to the grand prize! If you can answer these questions correctly, you will walk out of here with the new house, two new cars, the new wardrobe, and a cashier's check for One Million Dollars. All you need to do is quickly name all your past medical illnesses, when they occurred, who took care of you, what tests were done, what the results were, what your diagnoses were, how the illnesses were treated, and whether hospitalizations were required. While you're at it, throw in your early developmental history, your childhood illnesses, and list any bad reactions you have had to medications.

This sounds absurd; how can anyone be expected to remember all of this information off the top of their head without any warning or preparation? Yet, this type information, also known as the *Past Medical History* (PMH), is requested in a similar fashion all the time, especially when people meet a doctor for the first time. There must be a better way!

This chapter is about how to organize this voluminous information for your doctor before you come to the office. The PMH is an essential part of the medical evaluation because it creates the context for and may help explain your current symptoms. It is also plays an integral part in decisions about future treatments because some therapies are indicated or proscribed in the face of certain underlying medical conditions.

Prepare your past medical history *before* you see the doctor.

> Dr. Jones completed the requisition for an MRI (picture of the brain) for Mr. Jacobs, a 65-year-old man with headaches. Mr.

Jacobs has prepared a list of his past medical problems, including kidney stones and gallbladder disease.

So far so good, except for one *small* thing. Also on the list is a notation referring to a metal plate that was inserted into Mr. Jacob's head after incurring a head injury. Reviewing the list, Dr. Jones rips up his requisition and breathes a sigh of relief after realizing that performing an MRI would have been disastrous given the intense magnetic forces used in MRIs.

Considering all of the information your doctor needs to review, it is very easy to miss small but crucial aspects of your past medical history. Help your doctor remember the important facts about your background by maintaining an organized list and description of each medical problem.

Help your relatives go down in history.

> You accompany your Uncle Gordon, a 68-year-old man who suffered a stroke last year, to see a new doctor for a checkup. He is unable to speak and is brought in a wheelchair. He arrives for his first visit accompanied by an aide from the nursing home who is unfamiliar with his medical history.

There is just one problem. No one has prepared any information for the doctor. The doctor must call the nursing home, but he might end up waiting fifteen minutes on the line until he finds a staff member who is familiar with Mr. Gordon. The staff member will then have to sift through chart notes over the ensuing half-hour, but the prior medical history may still remain unclear. The doctor will probably request that copies of the notes to be sent to him, but now he must reschedule the visit when more information is available. What could be more frustrating? How can he possibly adequately evaluate and treat his patient?

Yes, it does take some effort to prepare a past medical history, but organizing this information ultimately saves time for everyone. The information serves as an ongoing record of the medical history and does not need to be recreated every time the person is seen by a new practitioner. You can use Form 3 to accomplish this.

Components of the Past Medical History (PMH)

The PMH is a summary of the major landmarks in your prior health, including both elements of illness and also good health, such as normal early development and pregnancy. If you prepare your PMH before seeing the doctor, it is not necessary to go into tremendous detail for each prior illness in the same way you did for the History of Present Illness. Give your doctor just enough information so that she can understand how active or dormant the particular problem is and how it affects your current health.

Here are some tips for preparing your PMH:

- **Adult Illnesses:** Mention any illnesses, surgeries, accidents, or injuries you incurred in the past. Also include any psychiatric difficulties.

- **Pregnancy:** Give enough detail for your doctor to use it as a reference in future gynecological or obstetrical health care.

- **Childhood illnesses and immunizations:** This can be very difficult to recall, but this information is worth getting from your prior doctors or from family members. Questions about childhood illnesses and past vaccinations will come up repeatedly when seeing new doctors or even on typical employee health forms.

- Tell your doctor how each problem affected you. For example, a bout with the flu in some people could be merely a severe cold, but for others it could land them in the hospital and unable to work or function at home during the recovery period.

For each of your medical problems, tell your doctor whether the problem persists, has resolved, or gotten better but you were left with complications. Note whether the doctor continues to follow that problem and, if so, how often is it checked?

The Problem List

Once each problem has been outlined in the PMH form, you can summarize each problem on one page and call it your *problem list*. Actually, doctors are supposed to keep such a list for you in your medical chart, but this is often not done. Therefore, it is very helpful to keep your own problem list, which can be used as a quick reference. This way, the important past and current problems can be addressed each time you see the doctor.

For example, a 50-year-old woman with multiple prior past medical problems often gets flustered when meeting the doctor. She often realizes when she returns home from an office visit that she forgot to address a minor, but still important, problem of an ulcer on her foot. Her problem list might look like the following:

- Diabetes mellitus
- Stroke
- Bronchitis

- Ulcer on foot
- Bad reaction to insulin, 1997
- Dizziness
- Allergy to penicillin
- Cataracts
- Memory problem
- Shaking of the hands

Referring to a problem list before and during the office visit will ensure that all your major concerns have been covered. In the next chapter, we will see how information about illnesses that run in families can greatly contribute to understanding your own medical symptoms and how it may even lead to a diagnosis.

FORM 3

Past Medical History

History of Birth and Early Development:

Were there any difficulties in the pregnancy when your mother was pregnant with you? _____

_____

Was your birth full-term? _____

Were you delivered with the use of forceps or cesarean section?_____

As far as you know, by what age were you walking? _____

By what age were you talking? _____

Handedness:

Are you right- or left-handed? _____

Allergies:

Do you have hay fever or specific bad reactions to foods or things in the environment? _____

_____

Summarize the names of any medications (including anesthesia) that have caused bad reactions, and list the details in the *Treatments Form*.

_____

_____

Pregnancy History:

How many times have you been pregnant? _____

How many pregnancies came to full term births?_____

How many pregnancies came to premature births? Provide additional information:_____

_____

How many pregnancies were aborted? Provide additional information: _____

_____

Were these pregnancies spontaneous abortions, induced, or elective? _____

_____

How many children are currently living? _____

Did you have any specific complications or problems during any pregnancies? If so, provide details. _____

_____

Was labor induced or spontaneous? _____

Were deliveries vaginal or cesarean? If cesarean why? _____

Did you have any postpartum problems, such as infection or phlebitis? _____

_____

Were there any problems for the baby immediately after birth, such as jaundice or infections? _____

_____

Childhood Illnesses:

List your history of:

	Year (if known)	Age (if known)
Measles	_____	_____
Rubella	_____	_____
Mumps	_____	_____

Whooping Cough	_____	_____
Chicken-pox	_____	_____
Rheumatic Fever	_____	_____
Scarlet Fever	_____	_____
Polio	_____	_____
Other	_____	_____

Immunizations:

Type of Vaccine	Date or Age it was Last Received	Any Bad Reactions?
Tetanus	_____	_____
Pertussis	_____	_____
Diphtheria	_____	_____
Polio	_____	_____
Measles	_____	_____
Rubella	_____	_____
Mumps	_____	_____
Influenza	_____	_____
Hepatitis B	_____	_____
Haemophilus Influenzae	_____	_____
Pneumococcus	_____	_____
Lyme	_____	_____
Chicken Pox (Varicella)	_____	_____
Other:	_____	_____
Other:	_____	_____
Other:	_____	_____

Adult Illnesses:

List all of the illnesses you have had as an adult—for example: high blood pressure, diabetes, asthma, heart disease, cancer, HIV, tuberculosis, prior surgeries, psychiatric difficulties, accidents, and injuries. Make multiple copies of this section of Form 3, if necessary, for multiple illnesses.

Name of the problem:_____

Date or age it originally began: _____

How did it begin or present itself? _____

_____

_____

Subsequently, what dates or ages did you experience recurrences or
worsening or the problem?_____

_____

What were some landmark events during the course of the illness; what
happened; did it resolve? _____

_____

What were the names of doctors or medical centers where you were treated
and the dates of any evaluations you received for this problem? _____

_____

_____

How was the problem diagnosed—for example: specific evaluation,
examination, or test? _____

What was the diagnosis?_____

What tests were performed? List the names of the tests, but fill in the
details on Form 5, *Prior Testing Results* (see page 43). _____

_____

_____

What were the most severe problems you experienced as a result of this
illness?_____

_____

_____

Currently, do you have any persistent complications or residual effects? _____

_____

_____

Prior treatments: List the names of prior treatments, but list the details on
Forms 6C and 6D (see pages 47 and 48). _____

_____

_____

List the names of your current treatments, but list the details on Forms 6A and 6B (see pages 46 and 47). _____

_____

_____

What is the current status of the illness? Do you have any persistent complications or residual effects? What follow-up are you receiving and are any future treatments planned? _____

_____

_____

Other comments: _____

_____

_____

CHAPTER 5

All in the Family—Your Family History

"John Fletcher's brother Phil was a month shy of turning 42 when a malignant tumor was found in his colon. John, who was only 39 at the time, had never given a whole lot of thought to his family medical history. Although he had never smoked, John was a good 20 pounds overweight and seldom exercised. After hearing the news about his brother, he became more curious about the high incidence of cancer in his family, particularly since his mother had died from ovarian cancer at the age of 62. As he started interviewing relatives about other family members, he learned that his maternal grandfather had died at the age of 32 from a tumor in the colon that was situated exactly where Phil's tumor was located. Thinking that he had inherited some of these same genes from his mother and grandfather, he made an appointment for a complete physical. Thankfully, he was given a clean bill of health. He now gets colon exams on a regular basis."

CAROL DAUS
Past Imperfect

This is an example of the importance of conducting an examination of the disorders that run in your family, which may have implications on your own current or future health. Here are some examples where knowledge of illnesses in the family can help clarify your own set of symptoms:

- Hereditary diseases that may be passed on from one generation to the next—for example, sickle cell disease and Huntington's chorea.

- Conditions that tend to run in families and raise the risk of getting the disease, such as heart disease and psychiatric illness, but where the role of specific genetic factors has not been worked out yet.

- Disorders that have a genetic component but that may also influence an individual's health through exposure to the abnormal behaviors or habits of the affected family member, such as manic-depression (bipolar disorder) and alcoholism.

- Striking physical characteristics in the family history that may suggest a diagnosis—for example, facial features in Down's syndrome or cleft palate.

- Information in the family history that leads the doctor to recommend screening of other family members for inheritable disorders. For example, a diagnosis of Fragile X syndrome may lead to genetic testing of females in the family to determine whether they are at risk for having sons with Fragile X.

- Information about ethnic background. This can be useful because certain genetic disorders tend to be more common in specific ethnic groups—for example, Tay-Sachs disease in Ashkenazi Jews or cystic fibrosis in Caucasian populations.
- Knowledge about illnesses that run in a family. This information does not always lead to the conclusion of an inherited disease because some illnesses can be contagious or the result of exposure to hazardous substances.[2]

You can help your doctor learn about your family's medical history by preparing Form 4 before you see the doctor.

Preparing your family history can help your doctor make a diagnosis.

Try not to get upset when preparing your family history. Sometimes, discussing illnesses that run in the family may bring up sad feelings as you recall those in the family who suffered or died from a particular disease. Sometimes these thoughts can be depressing or frightening, especially if the family member's symptoms remind you of your current problem. Having a family member with an illness may create fear that you will also contract it. It is best to discuss these feelings openly with your doctor.

In preparing your family history, it is worth mentioning illnesses such as:

- Cancer
- Diabetes
- Heart disease
- Strokes
- Colitis (inflammation of the gastrointestinal tract)
- High blood pressure
- Elevated cholesterol
- Neurologic conditions, such as Alzheimer's disease, Lou Gehrig's disease, multiple sclerosis, and hereditary peripheral nerve diseases

Your medical problem can be clarified not only by understanding symptoms experienced by you or your family, but also by reviewing the results of tests that have been previously performed in pursuit of your diagnosis. In the

2. *The Medical Interview: Mastering Skills for Clinical Practice* by J.L. Coulehan and M.R. Block. Philadelphia: F.A. Davis Company, 1997.

next chapter, we show you how to optimally organize your prior diagnostic workup information.

Family Medical History

Family Members

Include medical or psychiatric illnesses, striking physical characteristics, mental retardation, birth defects, miscarriages, or symptoms similar to ones you have experienced.

Relationship	If alive, current age	If deceased, age at time of death	Cause of death	Illnesses during lifetime	Age each illness began	Ethnicity
Mother						
Father						
Brother #1						
Brother #2						
Brother #3						

Sister #1					
Sister #2					
Sister #3					
Son #1					
Son #2					
Son #3					
Daughter #1					
Daughter #2					
Daughter #3					
Spouse					
Other(s)*					

*List other members of your extended family, such as grandparents, uncles, aunts, cousins, nieces, and nephews. Specify if they are on your father or mother's side.

CHAPTER 6

Put Yourself to the Test— Your Prior Diagnostic Workup

Has something similar to this happened to you?

> Dr. Carver is the third doctor you have seen for fainting episodes. You know you have had many prior tests and you recall being told about some kind of abnormality on a Holter monitor. You also recall that something was seen on either the CAT scan or MRI of your head, but you think that the doctors were not concerned about this finding. Dr. Carver is interested in seeing the reports and ideally would like to review many of the actual tests herself. However, you cannot remember the specific location where each test was performed and you only remember some of the names of the tests you had.

If this is *you*, do not feel alone. This is one of the most commonly encountered problems, in which the doctor must begin a fresh evaluation of a problem that has previously been investigated but for which no information is available. Dr. Carver needs to decide whether it is worth trying to track down each prior test, secretly dreading the thought of the numerous phone calls she will need to make to clarify the prior workup, and feeling paralyzed about proceeding with the investigation until she collects this important information. Given her pessimism about obtaining this information promptly, do not be surprised if she simply repeats a lot of tests, some perhaps unnecessarily.

Instead, let us say you were seeing Dr. Chang because of coughing episodes:

> You have kept a list of each of your prior tests and the date and place where each was performed. You requested a copy of each test result from your prior doctors and where possible you obtained actual copies of each test. Yes, you did have to take two hours off from work to go the X-ray facility and pick up an actual copy of the films. The chest X-ray was read as normal, but Dr. Chang inspects the actual films and feels that the quality is

really suboptimal. She repeats the X-rays, and good thing she did, because this time she sees a spot that needs to be worked up further.

Bravo! You have done much better this time. You greatly assisted your doctor by providing not only test results but in some cases the actual tests for the doctor to review. Dr. Chang was able to make an immediate assessment about the adequacy of the prior workup, and she made a prompt decision about further investigation. In the first circumstance, your diagnostic workup remained in limbo, but you may have saved your life the second time around.

In summary, your doctor needs to know about any prior tests that are related to your current medical problem. Without these test results, your doctor may postpone making decisions about diagnosis and treatment, and valuable time will be wasted collecting prior test results. A preferable alternative is to prepare as many test reports and, ideally, actual copies of tests before the office visit.

Form 5 provides an organized way of summarizing prior testing in preparation for review by the doctor. Make multiple copies of the following form and complete one for each test.

List each prior test in the order you received them, and use your discretion about which tests to include. For example, if a blood test is performed every month to check that anemia is not developing, it would not be worth listing every single blood test result; instead, cite only the few that had significant abnormalities and those taken recently.

Even if you have copies of the actual test to show the doctor, take the time to write the test results on the form. This will help organize the findings for your doctor to review. Even if you cannot understand the medical language used in the test reports, note that virtually all medical test reports conclude with a summary or impression. You can write this final summary on the form under *Results* and indicate that the full report is available for review by the doctor.

You are entitled to all your prior medical records in order to show them to any new doctor you consult. While the actual medical record belongs by law to the health care provider or medical center, you are entitled to a copy of the information in your medical record. The original record cannot be removed from the doctor's office or hospital, but you are entitled to receive copies by paying a reasonable fee. To obtain a copy of the record, you will be asked to sign a Release of Information form. This is actually a good thing, because it ensures that confidential medical information is not distributed to anyone without your permission.

The recently introduced Health Insurance Portability and Accountability Act (HIPAA) further establishes protections and safeguards for patient health information. It protects an individual's identifiable medical record, gives individuals the right to know who has or will see their medical records, allows patients to review and amend records, and reduces disclosure of health information to the minimum necessary. When you visit the doctor or sign a release of information form, you will likely be asked to sign papers that stipulate how the medical facility is compliant with HIPAA regulations and in what circumstances personal medical information can be revealed. Also, be aware that medical tests and other records in your medical evaluation are kept for at least seven years in doctors' offices and longer in medical centers. Medical tests and reports are also stored at the facilities where the test was performed. [3]

In the next chapter, we will learn how knowledge about responses to prior or current treatments can influence your doctor's thinking about your diagnosis as well as how it may change ideas for future treatments.

FORM 5

Prior Testing Results

Name of test: _____

What part of the body was tested: _____

Date of test: _____

Where the test was performed: _____

Results: _____

_____

_____

_____

Name of test: _____

What part of the body was tested: _____

Date of test: _____

Where the test was performed: _____

Results: _____

_____

_____

_____

3. *Making Informed Medical Decisions: Where to Look and How to Use What You Find* by N. Oster, L. Thomas and D. Joseff. Cambridge: O'Reilly, 2000

CHAPTER 7

Current and Prior Treatments

Bring a list of your medications and the dosages each time you see the doctor; do not assume she has this information.

> Mr. Bender learned the hard way that it was not a good idea to visit the doctor unprepared. He showed up at the doctor's office urgently asking for refills when he ran out of his blood pressure medications, but he did not bring his medication information. Dr. Burns had a notation in the records listing the name of the medication, but the dose was not listed. No problem; Dr. Burns simply told Mr. Bender to call in the information from home. But Mr. Burns got stuck in traffic and by the time he got home the office was closed. The next morning, he placed an urgent call to his doctor, but he had already missed a dose.

Doctors see this problem all the time. Sometimes the dose a person thinks he is supposed to take does not match the medical records. At other times, the doses may have been changed in between office visits and there is no documentation of the new dose in the medical records. In order to make sure that you and your doctor know what medications you are taking and the correct dosages, keep a list of them on Form 6A and bring in the actual pill containers.

Out with the old, in with the new!

> Ms. Marcus was looking for a miracle. Perhaps world-famous Dr. Warren could find the cure for her chronic migraine headaches. She had tried so many medications, some of which worked a little bit but had side effects, and others that caused side effects and didn't work at all. Dr. Warren proposed that she start on a medication called amitriptyline. However, Ms. Marcus vaguely recalls having tried this medication in the past, although she is not sure about this, and she certainly does not recall when she tried it, how much she was given, or why she

stopped taking it. Dr. Warren proposed propranolol or topira-mate, but Ms. Marcus thinks she may have been on these medications before. In fact, short of divine intervention, we are not likely to witness any miracles today, because Dr. Warren does not know where to start in treating Ms. Marcus.

If you do not come prepared with the names and details about your prior medications, your doctor is going to have difficulty devising a treatment plan. Take the time to prepare *before* you see the doctor. Get your old records and talk to anyone who can help you recall these vital bits of information. Form 6C will help you organize this information about prior medications and other types of treatments.

The devil is in the details!

Tell your doctor exactly *when* you take each medication. Timing sometimes makes a world of difference in the effectiveness of a drug.

> Ms. Thompson was evaluated by Dr. Sanders for diabetes-related nerve pains in her feet. She was recently prescribed gabapentin but it is not working. Is it time to move on to another treatment? Not so fast. Reviewing when the pills are taken reveals that she is taking gabapentin at exactly the same time as her antacid, and antacids can interfere with the absorption of gabapentin into the body. So, instead of jumping to a new treatment, the doctor decided to stagger the times when she takes each medication. On the following visit, Ms. Thompson indicated that her pain is greatly improved.

Don't just do something, stand there!

If your doctor hears that you were on a previous medication and it did not work, the natural inclination is to try a different treatment approach. However, sometimes it is better to stop and consider more of the details about your prior treatments.

> Ms. Kelly was also evaluated by Dr. Warren for chronic migraines. She has maintained detailed records of all the treatments she has received. Using this record, Dr. Warren noted that amitriptyline was started at 50 mg. per day and was stopped after only four days because she became very sleepy. Dr. Warren prescribed amitriptyline again, but only 10 mg. before going to sleep each night. Using this prescription, she did

not get sleepy during the day and her headaches improved quite a bit. Dr. Warren gradually increased the dose to 20 mg. per day, which stopped the headaches.

One of the most common errors doctors make is jumping from one treatment to another without giving each treatment a fair trial. After a while, this can mean that there are no treatments left to try. Giving your doctor details about your prior treatments can help reduce these gymnastics.

Sometimes a drug will never be tried again because a side effect occurred. However, some side effects can be temporary. If your doctor knows that an effective drug was used for only a short time, it may be worth trying again and waiting to see if the side effects subside.

For example, you may ask, "When I got my new hand drill, it came with many warnings as to how to avoid getting an electric shock. How come I did not get any warning about getting dizzy and stomach aches when I got my new prescription from the doctor?"

We are always amazed to hear how often doctors prescribe a treatment without reviewing the side effects. In Chapter 12, the questions you should ask your doctor when a treatment is recommended are reviewed, even if the doctor does not volunteer this information. By the way, do not forget to mention nontraditional treatments, such as acupuncture, chiropractic manipulations, and other alternative or complementary medicine techniques, that you have received; your doctor needs to know about them, too.

So far, we have spent a lot of time focusing on your symptoms, but what about the effect these symptoms have on your quality of life? In the next chapter, we will explore this issue and find ways to make your doctor better appreciate how well or how poorly you are coping with a medical problem.

FORM 6A

Current Medication Treatments

Indicate the following for each medication you are currently taking:

Name of medication: _____

When did you begin taking this medication? _____

Total dose of medication per day: _____

How many mg. per pill and how is it given throughout the day: _____

Were you ever on a higher dose than currently?_____

If so, why was it reduced? _____

Is the medication helping? If so, in what way? _____
_____

Do you experience any side effects? _____
_____

Do you take the medication with food or on an empty stomach? _____

Do you take the medication every day or only when needed?_____

List any non-medication treatments you are currently receiving on Form 6B.

FORM 6B

Current Non-Medication Treatments

Non-medication treatments include acupuncture, chiropractic treatments, massage, biofeedback, and other alternative or complementary medicine techniques.

Name of treatment: _____

When did you begin receiving this treatment? _____

Describe the treatment. How is it given? _____
_____

Is the treatment helping? If so, in what way? _____
_____

Do you experience any side effects? _____
_____

FORM 6C

Prior Medications

Complete the following information for each prior treatment:

Name of medication or treatment: _____

When was it started? _____

When was it stopped?_____

Why was it stopped? _____

Was it effective? _____

What was the highest dose ever used? _____

Did you experience any side effects? _____

_____

Please also list non-medication treatments used in the past on Form 6D.

Prior Non-Medication Treatments

Non-medication treatments include acupuncture, chiropractic treatments, massage, biofeedback, or other alternative or complementary medicine techniques.

Name of treatment: _____

When did you received this treatment: _____

Describe the treatment. How was it given?_____

_____

_____

Did the treatment help? If so, in what way?_____

_____

_____

Did you experience any side effects? _____

_____

CHAPTER 8

Beyond the Facts and Figures –
Your Psychosocial History

When 58-year-old Mr. Hoffman went to see Dr. Anderson, the doctor told him how pleased he was that Mr. Hoffman's bronchitis and emphysema had not worsened. "The medications are working and you are doing very well," Dr. Anderson said. But Mr. Hoffman did not understand how the doctor could say this. After all, because of his lung disease, he cannot go out of the house, he cannot work, and he feels depressed most of the time. In fact, Mr. Hoffman does not share the doctor's optimism at all and often wonders whether life is even worth living.

How is possible that the doctor and the patient have arrived at such completely different conclusions about Mr. Hoffman's condition? One reason is that although the doctor has focused on symptoms, exam findings, and tests, he has ignored the effects of the illness on Mr. Hoffman's life. In doing so, he has neglected an essential component of the medical evaluation. In order to address these concerns, the doctor should have asked a series of questions that would elicit his patient's *psychosocial history*, enabling him to go beyond facts and figures about symptoms and problems, and learn more of his patient's personal information or, in essence, the answer to the question, "Who are you?" The psychosocial history delves into many facets of your current and prior life experiences. It puts the raw data of symptoms and signs into the context of a real person living a real life. Sometimes, psychosocial distress may be the real reason for seeing the doctor, or it may be the cause of or contribute to symptoms described earlier in the history. When time is devoted to discussing the psychosocial history, the bond between doctor and patient is strengthened.

Although the doctor may not be the best equipped professional in terms of knowledge or resources to remedy psychosocial difficulties, he is in the best position to screen for these kinds of problems and then make recommendations where needed for further assistance. For example, having identified clues to possible depression, the doctor may recommend that other health care providers, such as social workers, psychologists, and psychiatrists, become involved.

Although your psychosocial history can rarely be adequately assessed by merely reading your written responses, the questions in Form 7A will give you a flavor of the kinds of information that the doctor wants to know. Because this subject deserves more thoughtful consideration, being aware of these questions before the doctor's visit provides the chance to carefully think about these issues.

The initial portion of Form 7A deals with your current living situation and relationships. Illness affects not only the person who is sick, but family and colleagues as well. The doctor is not only interested in the dry facts about relationships, but also how others are reacting to the illness. This portion of the psychosocial interview also helps the doctor screen for domestic physical or emotional neglect or violence.

The psychosocial history also delves into how the medical condition has affected your life. As in this example, a doctor may consider his medical efforts a complete success, while you may have a completely different point of view. You may think, "The doctor does not understand; these symptoms are ruining my life!"

Tell your doctor whether you are dealing with the illness alone or whether there are others who provide emotional support. Are there strong relationships among family members that can help you cope with illness, or are there conflicts that interfere with your healing? If you have limited mobility, who is helping you? Who is preparing your meals? If you are not independent, who is helping you take care of your financial matters? Looking into these areas is more than expressing sympathy; part of the doctor's role is to work with social agencies to facilitate these other health care needs.

> "A doctor…would inform me that I had a progressive, degenerative, and incurable neurologic disorder; one that I may have been living with for as long as a decade before suspecting there might be anything wrong…. Coping with the relentless assault and the accumulating damage is not easy. Nobody would ever choose to have this visited on them. Still, this unexpected crisis forced a fundamental life decision: adopt a siege mentality or embark on a journey. What it was—courage? acceptance? wisdom?—that finally allowed me to go down the second road

(after spending a few disastrous years on the first) was unquestionably a gift—and absent this neurophysiologic catastrophe, I would never have opened it or been so profoundly enriched. That's why I consider myself a lucky man."

MICHAEL J. FOX
Lucky Man: A Memoir

Religious and Cultural Issues

In addition to any current psychosocial issues, the doctor learns about you by asking questions about your prior background (see second portion of Form 7A). A question about where you are originally from relates to the fact that there are many potential cultural differences in the way individuals interpret and deal with illness—for example, in some cultures it may be taboo to acknowledge certain types of illness or their treatments. Knowing the educational background of the patient can help the doctor decide how to best explain things to you. Even knowing about leisure activities reveals a great deal about you and can lead to strategies for leading as normal a life as possible, even in the face of illness.

My doctor is sending me for surgery, but my religion forbids me from having a blood transfusion.

Information about religious beliefs is useful in the context of medical illness, because religion often plays a crucial role in a person's reactions to illness and their ability to cope with illness. Certain religions forbid blood transfusions or other medical interventions. Your doctor will need to revise your treatments if your religion has specific prohibitions.

Occupation, Exposures, and Finances

Your doctor also needs to know about your work and income. A work history is important since any job, with its associated stresses and hazards, could affect your health. Understanding what you were able to do in the workplace, or what you are currently doing, helps the doctor assess how disabled you may be and shape goals for your future rehabilitation. The doctor can learn about your quality of life, relationships, and income by inquiring about the nature of your work, how well you are compensated, and how well you get along with others on the job.

The psychosocial history also includes possible exposures to toxins that may have occurred in the workplace. However, if the doctor suspects toxic exposures, a much more detailed history is needed. If this applies to you, be prepared to provide a chronological account of all jobs held, the nature and degree of exposure to toxins with each position held, the dates each job was held, and when the jobs were terminated. Try to recall what protective measures were instituted with each job, whether the toxic exposures were constant or intermittent, and how close you were to the source of the toxins. The work history also examines possible hazards such as risks for accidents, or injury.

Sexuality

One of the most significant ways that illness affects individuals is in their sexual relationships.

> Janet became extremely depressed when, six months after her second marriage, she found herself unable to have an orgasm during sex. She did not think of this response as a medical problem, but even if she had, she would have been too embarrassed to mention it to her doctor.
>
> It was only by accident that she began to suspect that the cause of her sexual difficulty was her blood pressure medicine, methyldopa (Aldomet®). By a stroke of luck, she developed a stomach virus and temporarily stopped taking her Aldomet®. As she recovered from the virus, her libido and ability to have orgasms returned. But her sexual problems returned when she went back on the Aldomet®.
>
> A few experiments of not taking her medicine for a few days and then having sex increased her growing suspicions, and her doctor confirmed the link between the drug and her sex life when she finally asked him.
>
> The doctor inquired, perhaps rather naively, "Why didn't you tell me about this when your sexual problems first started?"
>
> She was too nice to respond, "Why didn't you inform me about the possible side effects?"
>
> RICHARD N. PODELL AND WILLIAM PROCTOR
> *When Your Doctor Does Not Know Best: Medical Mistakes that Even the Best Doctors Make and How to Protect Yourself*

Despite the purported openness advanced by everyday exposure to issues of sexuality in the media, many doctors and patients find it difficult to discuss sexual health openly during the typical medical encounter. This is unfortunate, since sexual problems are very common and often remain undisclosed. Fortunately, it is becoming more common for doctors to be exposed to these topics in medical school and residency programs. Nevertheless, some doctors still feel uncomfortable bringing up these issues. In such circumstances, people need to be proactive about raising these types of concerns.

The Review of Systems form also touches on sexual dysfunction, but the psychosocial history delves further into issues related to sexual satisfaction and relationships (see Form 9, page 71). It is not necessary to write out the answers to the questions on Form 7B. If you prefer, you can just think about these questions and your possible answers, in order to discuss them with your doctor if you choose to.

FORM 7A

Your Psychosocial History

What kind of residence do you live in—for example, a private home or a supervised facility? _____

_____

Who do you live with? _____

_____

Are you single, married, divorced, or separated? _____

Have you previously been married, divorced, or separated? _____

_____

Describe your most important current relationships? _____

_____

_____

_____

What are some of the good and bad aspects of these relationships? _____

_____

_____

_____

Are you or have you been satisfied with your sexual relationships? _____

Do you or have you had any difficulties in this area and, if so, what kind? ___

_____

_____

_____

How has your medical problem affected your activities of daily living, work, relationships, and mood? _____

_____

_____

_____

How are you coping with your medical problems? _____

_____

_____

Who is available to give you emotional support or, if needed, transportation to the doctor, and arrange for your financial needs? _____

_____

_____

Important Experiences:

Where are you from originally? _____

What is your highest level of education and where did you go to school? ___

_____

What do you do for recreation? What are your hobbies? _____

_____

_____

Religion and Beliefs:

Do your religious beliefs affect how you allow yourself to be treated medically? _____

Occupation/Exposures/Finances:

Are you employed? _____

What is your main source of income or support? _____

_____

What do you currently do for a living and what have you done in the past? ___

_____

_____

If married, what does your spouse do for a living? _____

_____

How do you like your work—for example, the nature of your work, the hours, compensation, and working with others? If not currently working, how did you like your work in the past? _____

_____

_____

_____

_____

How would you describe your level of physical and/or emotional stress as related to your work? _____

_____

Is your work associated with significant risks for injuries or accidents? _____

_____

Has your work entailed any repetitive movements or major lifting? _____

Do you think any of your symptoms or medical problems are related to work? _____

_____

What hours do you work and how do you feel about your work schedule? ___

_____

Sexuality[4]

General Questions

What is your sexual preference? _____

Has any current illness has affected sexual functioning? _____

Describe the nature and number of sexual partners: _____

_____

_____

_____

Have you engaged in sexual behaviors that are at high risk for sexually-transmitted diseases, such as intravenous drug abuse, relations with homosexual or bisexual men, prostitutes, or unknown partners? _____

_____

What methods of birth control have you been using? _____

What worries or questions do you have about sexual diseases or sex in general?_____

_____

_____

For men:

Have you had any difficulties attaining or maintaining an erection? _____

Do you experience premature ejaculation? _____

Does ejaculation occur outward or inward? _____

For women:

Do you experience pain during intercourse? _____

Do you have problem attaining orgasm or have difficulties with arousal or lubrication? _____

_____

4. Adapted in part from *The Sexual History* by Williams S. in *The Medical Interview, Clinical Care, Education, and Research* by M.J. Lipkin S.M. Putnam, and A Lazare, Editors. New York: Springer-Verlag, 1995:235-250)

In clarifying sexual problems in a psychosocial evaluation, you can expect questions such as:

When did problems begin? _____

Are the problems specific to one partner? _____

How are you and your partner reacting to the problem? _____

_____

_____

How was your prior sexual functioning? _____

_____

_____

Earlier in life, did you experience painful or emotionally traumatic sexual experiences? _____

_____

_____

_____

Do you experience any conflicts about sexual preference? _____

_____

_____

Your medical history is not only about illness but also aspects of your lifestyle that promote or prevent future illness. We will learn about this in the next chapter.

CHAPTER 9

Your Current and Future Health

Medical Economics

> "He did not come down on me real hard. I did not feel like I had been sent to the vice principal's office and he was wagging a finger in my face saying, 'You better do this' or 'you better do that.'
>
> Instead, he came across like he was a very knowledgeable friend. He said that I had a pretty high risk of heart attack or stroke, and that if nothing changed I'd probably have to go on insulin. 'You're still a pretty young man. Do you want to see these things happen?'
>
> When I said that of course I did not want that, he told me that we could prevent it. We had a lot of work to do, but it could be done. It was not impossible. From then on, I was on a diet, I started walking every day, and I came in to his office every two weeks. He would talk to me, encourage me, keep me going. That helped a lot."
>
> MIKE MAGEE AND MICHAEL D'ANTONIO
> *Patience for Patients, in The Best Medicine*

Dr. Clark never thought about asking about alcohol use when 45-year-old Mr. Baker appeared intermittently over the years for treatment of a bad cough or headache. That's why Dr. Clark was especially surprised when Mr. Baker presented with vomiting and swelling of the abdomen. This time, taking a more thorough history revealed that Mr. Baker drinks seven beers a day. In fact, alcoholism has led to loss of his job and the breakup of his marriage.

Most of this book is about discussing disease symptoms with your doctor. Yet the medical evaluation is not only concerned with current and past illness; it is also about identifying risk factors for future medical problems and injuries. Therefore, your doctor needs to know if you smoke, drink, use drugs, have a poor diet, or do not exercise enough. The doctor also needs to know if there are any other problems that need to be addressed. We have prepared Form 8 for this purpose.

Many people who abuse alcohol or drugs are reluctant to acknowledge or share this type of information. Many people with an alcohol problem are not able to confront their illness, and even those who do are often reluctant to admit to an alcohol problem. Remember that your doctor's interest in this issue is not to be a cop or judge, but rather to understand how these problems can affect your health.

My doctor devoted the whole office visit to discussing my sore throat, but I am upset about being very overweight and we did not even discuss this.

Today, many Americans are battling the problem of being overweight, which can cause medical complications such as diabetes, heart disease, high blood pressure, and stroke. Alternatively, insufficient body weight may be a sign of disease or abnormal diet. Knowing about diet can help the doctor devise recommendations for preventing future weight-related consequences. Unfortunately, questions about nutrition are often neglected in typical medical interviews, and having questions about it, such as those in Form 8, keeps it high on the agenda.

Many of us also do not exercise enough (Author A.E. pleads guilty to this charge), yet exercise is very important for maintaining good health. Your doctor can prescribe an appropriate exercise regimen by knowing your current exercise habits, and he will know what is advisable if you have any medical condition. Good preventive health care also involves inquiries about safety habits—for example, using a helmet when riding a bicycle or applying sunscreen to reduce the chances of skin cancer.

The final portion of Form 8 deals with common screening tests that are administered in order to look for diseases, such as tuberculosis, colon cancer, irregular heart rhythms, lung tumors, cervical cancer, and breast tumors. Other tests performed by the doctor can be added to the list. By keeping an ongoing record of these screening tests and updating the doctor, future testing can be ordered at the appropriate intervals.

You are almost done preparing your medical history, but did we forget anything? In the next chapter, we will learn a way to cover all those remaining loose ends.

Current Health Form

Tobacco:

Do you currently use tobacco? _____

If so, do you smoke or chew tobacco? _____

How much do you smoke per day? _____

How long have you been a smoker? _____

If you do not use tobacco now, but you were a former user, how long ago
did you quit? _____

How long did you use tobacco before you quit? _____

Alcohol:

Do you currently drink alcohol? _____

How much do you drink in a given day or week? _____

Have you ever had a drinking problem? _____

When was your last drink? _____

Do you have blackouts, seizures, injuries, or other problems due to
drinking? _____

_____

Have you had problems with work or relationships due to drinking? _____

_____

Drug Use:

Do you use illegal drugs? _____

If so, what types of drugs, how much, and how often? _____

_____

How long have you been using illegal drugs? _____

If you do not use illegal drugs currently but did in the past, how long ago
did you quit? _____

How long were you using illegal drugs before you quit? _____

Exercise and Diet:

What kind of exercise do you perform? _____

How often do you exercise and for how long have you been exercising on a regular basis? _____

_____

What does your typical diet consist of? _____

_____

_____

Are there any restrictions on your diet? _____

Do you use dietary supplements? _____

If so, which ones and in what amounts? _____

How much caffeine do you consume per day? _____

Safety Measures:

Do you wear seatbelts? _____

Do you wear a bicycle helmet if you ride a bike? _____

Do you use sunblock regularly? _____

Have you receiving the following screening tests?

Name of Test	Last Time Checked	Results
Tuberculin	_____	_____
Cholesterol	_____	_____
Stool check for blood	_____	_____
Electrocardiogram	_____	_____
Chest X-ray	_____	_____
For women: Pap smear	_____	_____
For women: Mammogram	_____	_____
Other:	_____	_____
Other:	_____	_____

CHAPTER 10

Did We Forget Anything? –
The Review of Systems

Medical Economics

You can help your doctor determine if there are other issues in your medical history that need to be addressed by completing the Review of Systems (ROS) form. The ROS is like a vacuum cleaner picking up all the crumbs that were missed in the previous forms. It consists of a series of brief questions about each system of the body. Asking these questions helps identify medical problems that were not previously discussed and may bring out a few more clues that clarify the main problems. Form 9 is an example of typical questions comprising an ROS.

> Ms. Carter, a 42-year-old woman with recent fluttering sensations in her chest, was very glad that Dr. Reynolds went through a Review of Systems. That is because after they were done talking about the chest symptoms, the ROS picked up the fact that Ms. Carter is going to the bathroom very frequently to urinate. She did not give this problem much attention, but Dr. Reynolds was concerned enough to order a urine test, which showed that she had a nasty urinary tract infection. Ms. Carter would not have received very badly needed antibiotic treatment, if not for the Review of Symptoms.

Don't get lost in the forest.

Reviewing the ROS with the doctor in a reasonable time frame can be difficult because it has to cover so many possible symptoms. That is why you should report only those symptoms that are significant. A significant symptom is usually one that occurs frequently, is chronic, or is severe. Do not emphasize every symptom that you have *ever* experienced; use your judgment and discretion. After all, any of us could think of a positive symptom, if we think back far enough; this is not the purpose of the ROS. Medical interviews with positive symptoms in every area lead to the history losing its focus and the doctor and patient getting lost in a forest of details.

ROS during the physical examination.

Some doctors prefer to complete the ROS while they perform the physical examination by asking questions as they examine each body part. Do not get scared; this does not mean the doctor has discovered something serious when examining a particular part of your body; the doctor is simply using the examination to remember questions that need to be asked about each body system.

Preparing and understanding the ROS.

If you prepare responses on the ROS Form before the office visit, the doctor can use it as an efficient way to screen for important problems. The doctor may ask for further details about the symptoms you mention in order to clarify whether they are significant.

The ROS may need to be postponed in some circumstances, such as emergencies or where time has to be spent mostly on the *History of Present Illness*. If the doctor rattles off a list of symptoms when performing the ROS and you do not understand what she is asking, make sure you ask for the question to be clarified.

Now that you are done preparing your medical history, it is time to learn why your doctor taps you with a hammer, squeezes your belly, and shines lights in your eyes. The physical examination will be discussed in the next chapter.

Review of Systems[5]

General:

What is your usual weight? _____

Have there been any recent changes in your weight? _____

Are you experiencing any weakness, fatigue or fever? _____

Skin:

Do you have any rashes, lumps, sores, itching, dryness, color change, or changes in hair or nails? _____

Head:

Do you have any headaches, head injuries, dizziness, or lightheadedness? ___

_____

Eyes:

Do you have good eyesight? _____

Do you wear glasses or contact lenses? _____

When was your last eye examination? _____

Do you have any eye pain, redness, excessive tearing, double vision, blurred vision, spots, suspects, flashing lights, glaucoma, or cataracts? _____

_____

Ears:

How is your hearing? _____

Do you have any drainage from your ears, ringing noises, or spinning sensations? _____

_____

5. Adapted in part from *Comprehensive History: Adult Patient*. In: *Bates' Guide to Physical Examination and History Taking* by L.S. Bickley and R.A. Hoekelman, Editors. 7th Ed. New York: Lippincott, 1999:35-39.

Nose and Sinuses:

Do you have frequent colds, nasal stuffiness, discharge, itching, hay fever, nose bleeds, or sinus trouble? _____

_____

Mouth and Throat:

What is the condition of your teeth and gums? _____

_____

Have you had bleeding gums or mouth sores? _____

_____

Have you had a sore tongue, dry mouth, frequent sore throats, hoarseness, or trouble swallowing? _____

_____

Do you have dentures and if so how well do they fit? _____

When was your last dental examination? _____

Neck:

Do you have any lumps, swollen glands, goiter, pain, or stiffness in your neck? _____

_____

Breasts:

Do you have any lumps, pain or discomfort, nipple discharge? _____

_____

Do you have any bleeding, tenderness or swelling? _____

_____

Do you perform self-examinations? _____

Respiratory:

Do you have any cough, sputum and if so what color and how much? _____

_____

Do you have any coughing up of blood, shortness of breath, wheezing, asthma, bronchitis, emphysema, pneumonia, tuberculosis, or pleurisy? _____

_____

When was your last chest X-ray? _____

Heart:

Do you have any heart trouble, high blood pressure, rheumatic fever, heart murmurs, chest pain or discomfort, such as tightness, pressure, or heaviness?

_____

_____

Do you have any palpitations, shortness of breath, shortness of breath when sitting or standing erect, shortness of breath suddenly at night, or swelling in your feet? _____

_____

Gastrointestinal:

How is your appetite? _____

Do you have any trouble swallowing, heartburn, nausea, vomiting, regurgitation, belching, vomiting of blood, or indigestion? _____

_____

_____

What is the frequency of your bowel movements and the color and consistency of your stools? _____

_____

Do you have any problems with gas or cramping? _____

Do you have any problems with swelling or fullness of your belly?_____

_____

Has there been any change in your bowel habits, rectal bleeding, black tarry stools, hemorrhoids, constipation, diarrhea, abdominal pain, food intolerance, excessive belching, passing of gas, or jaundice? _____

_____

Liver and Gallbladder:

Have you had any liver or gallbladder trouble, jaundice (yellow skin or eyes), pale or white stools, or hepatitis? _____

Urinary:

How often do you urinate? _____

Do you have excessively frequent urination, the need to urinate in the middle of the night, burning or pain on urination, blood in the urine, urgency, a reduced force or caliber of the urinary stream, trouble starting, or stopping or holding the urine, dribbling, urinary infections, or stones? _____

_____

_____

Genital – Male:

Do you have any hernias, discharge from or sores on the penis, pus or drip from the penis, painful or swollen testicles, history of sexually transmitted (venereal) diseases and the treatments? _____

_____

_____

What is your sexual preference? _____

Describe your level of sexual interest, function, satisfaction, birth control methods, condom use, and any related problems: _____

_____

_____

Have you been exposed to HIV? _____

Genital – Female:

At what age did you begin to have your period? _____

How regular are your periods. What is their frequency and how long do they last? How much do you bleed? Do you bleed between periods or after intercourse? _____

_____

When was your last menstrual period? Did you have any pain or premenstrual tension during your period? _____

_____

Do you have any vaginal discharge or itching? _____

If applicable, at what age did you go into menopause and what were your menopausal symptoms? _____

Did you have postmenopausal bleeding? _____

If you were born before 1971, were you ever exposed to DES (diethylstil-bestrol) due to your mother's use of this drug during pregnancy with you?

_____

Do you have any discharge, itching, sores, lumps, sexually transmitted diseases, or treatments for these problems? _____

Describe the number of pregnancies, the nature of the deliveries, the number of abortions (spontaneous and induced), and any complications you may have had as the result of being pregnant: _____

_____

_____

_____

What birth control methods do you use? _____

What is your sexual preference? _____

Describe your level of sexual interest, function, satisfaction, birth control methods, and any related problems: _____

_____

Do you have any pain during sexual intercourse? _____

Have you been exposed to HIV? _____

Peripheral Vascular:

Do you have any pain in your calves during walking, leg cramps, varicose veins, or past clots in the veins? _____

Do you have cold hands or feet? _____

Musculoskeletal:

Do you have any muscle or joint pains, stiffness, arthritis, limitation of movement, neck or backache, or arm or leg pains? _____

If so, describe the nature of the symptoms, such as any swelling, redness, pain, tenderness, stiffness, weakness, or limitation of motion or activity: ____

_____

_____

Neurologic:

Do you experience any fainting, blackouts, seizures, weakness, paralysis, numbness or loss of sensation, trouble speaking, trouble walking or with balance or coordination, tingling or feeling of pins and needles, tremors or other involuntary movements? _____

_____

_____

Do you have any difficulty sleeping? _____

Do you have any problems with thinking or your memory? _____

Blood:

Do you have any anemia, easy bruising or bleeding, or past transfusions or any reactions to them? _____

Have you been unusually pale recently? _____

Endocrine (Glands):

Do you have any thyroid trouble, extreme discomfort from heat or cold, diabetes, excessive sweating, thirst, hunger, or urination? _____

Do you feel hot or cold all the time? _____

Have you had any unusual weight gain or weight loss? _____

Have there been any major changes in your general appearance? _____

_____

Psychiatric:

Do you have any nervousness, tension, depression or anxiety, memory difficulties, frequent bad dreams, frightening thoughts, feelings as if others are out to get you or that others are controlling your thoughts? _____

_____

_____

CHAPTER II

Let's Get Physical—
The Physical Examination [6]

"When we arrived at a private entrance, two doctors were waiting at the end of a long hall. They were relieved to see me walk. This indicated that I had no paralysis in my legs.

Dr. Gold asked, 'Show me your teeth.' I bared my teeth as I have done in so many of my movies. What I did not know was that my right lip drooped down, covering my teeth at that side of my mouth. It was a sure sign of a stroke. I could understand everything the doctor said, but I could not talk."

KIRK DOUGLAS
My Stroke of Luck

The physical examination is the next step in the diagnostic process. While the medical interview is designed to bring out information about symptoms, the objective information brought out by the examination is called *signs*. Having narrowed down the list of diagnostic possibilities by taking a careful history, the physical examination is performed to look for signs that go for or against the suspected diagnoses. For example, if the doctor suspects liver disease as the cause of vomiting, finding yellow discoloration of the skin (jaundice) and an enlarged liver supports this diagnosis, although it does not necessarily exclude other disorders. Just as a single answer to a question during the medical interview does not make the diagnosis, signs on examination do not tend to absolutely rule in or rule out any disease. Sometimes the absence of a finding is just as important as a positive finding. So if a joint problem is suspected as the cause for pain in a limb, finding a normal joint with full range of motion, without swelling or tenderness, would discourage that diagnosis.

The nature of the physical examination performed by your doctor varies according to the nature of the problem being investigated, the purpose of the visit, and the specialty of the doctor. On some occasions, a more focused exam is appropriate; at other times, a more comprehensive screening exam is indicated. Therefore the failure of your doctor to perform every aspect of the exam

6. Adapted in part from *Physical Examination*. In: *Bates' Guide to Physical Examination and History Taking*, L.S. Bickley and R.A. Hoekelman RA, Editors, 7th Ed. New York: Lippincott, 1999:129-136.

listed here does not necessarily imply that the exam was incomplete; some parts of the examination may be unrelated to the specific question at hand. While it is beyond the scope of this book to review the methods and reasoning behind every element of the physical examination, understanding some of the highlights of the exam is helpful in preparing to visit the doctor.

Components of the Physical Examination

The astute doctor wastes no time in making observations. Even as early as the interview process, the doctor can make important observations even without laying a hand on the person. During this general inspection, obvious abnormalities in appearance may be apparent. For example, a person may look very distracted, may have obvious alcohol on the breath, or have an obvious deformity of a body part.

The formal physical examination usually begins with examination of what are called *vital signs*. These include temperature, pulse, blood pressure, and rate of respiration. This is often supplemented by measurement of height and weight.

Body Temperature

Elevated temperature (fever) occurs during infections, inflammations, or conditions that cause abnormalities in our internal thermostats. Very low temperature can occur with extreme exposure to cold or when the body is in shock.

Heart Rate

The pulse is the heart rate, which tends to be lower in athletes or as a result of certain medications, such as beta-blockers. Elevated pulse rate occurs with exercise and exertion as a compensation for low blood pressure, in response to certain medications, in overactive thyroid conditions, or in persons with anemia.

Blood Pressure

Blood pressure is measured by inflating a cuff known as a *sphygmomanometer* around the upper arm to the point that it compresses the blood flow through an artery. The cuff has a pressure gauge attached to it. The bell portion of a stethoscope is placed in the fold of the elbow above where the artery is. As the cuff pressure is slowly released, the pressure at the level where the first sound begins to be heard is known as the *systolic* pressure. As the cuff pressure continues to be released, the sounds of the pulse continue and then trail off. The pressure at which the last sound is heard is called the *diastolic* pressure. Blood pressure is usually expressed as the systolic blood pressure over the diastolic pressure. Your doctor is interested not only in the absolute blood pressure readings, but also how it compares to your prior readings. Elevation in blood pressure is often unassociated with symptoms, but it can cause many bodily complications, including damage to the heart and the blood vessels of many organs. Extremely low blood pressure can occur in states of shock. To exclude excessively low blood pressure, it is useful to have the blood pressure checked while standing as well as sitting.

Sometimes blood pressure can be falsely elevated when it is taken at the doctor's office and is not truly representative of what it is normally. If your blood pressure is elevated, make sure it is checked several times with a proper-sized blood pressure cuff and, if possible, measure it at home as well.

Respiratory Rate

Increased respiratory rate occurs normally during exertion, but also during problems with insufficient oxygen in the body as may be seen with problems in the lung or heart. Severely decreased respiratory rate can occur with major brain problems.

Facial Features

The examination now focuses on individual body parts and usually begins with the head. The doctor begins with observing the structure of the facial features. He may tap lightly on the forehead or cheeks to see if these areas are painful as may be seen with an underlying inflammation of the sinuses.

The Eyes

Examination of the outer eye includes the colored, round area in the middle called the *iris*, the black circle within it called the *pupil* and the white area called the *sclera*, which is covered by a transparent covering called the *conjunctiva*. Abnormalities can occur with any of these structures. For example, inflammation of the iris is called *iritis*, a condition that can occur as a part of an autoimmune illness. Yellow discoloration of the sclera (jaundice) can occur with severe liver disease. Pupils that are unequal in size can occur as a result of eye drops or may be due to neurologic problems. In conjunctivitis, the conjunctiva is red and inflamed.

Using an *ophthalmoscope*, an instrument that shines a light into and through the pupil, the doctor can inspect the *retina* (back layer of the eye). Abnormalities in the appearance of the blood vessels, such as abnormal narrowing or clots within the vessels, can give clues about diseases, such as high blood pressure, diabetes, or the risk of developing a stroke. Inspection of the ending of the nerve supplying the eye (optic nerve) at the retina can detect increased pressure in the brain — for example, from brain tumors or other masses.

The Ears

Examination of the ear is performed with an *otoscope*, which shines a light on the ear drum (the *tympanic membrane*). The doctor looks for any signs of redness or swelling that would suggest infection (*otitis media*). The doctor also checks for drainage from the ear.

The Nose

Inspection of the nose involves assessment of the mucous membranes; examination of the mouth includes review of the health of the teeth, the tongue and the oral mucous membranes to assess for abnormal growths. Redness or pus in the back of the throat suggests infection.

The Neck

In the neck exam, the doctor checks to see if movement of the head forward and backwards is stiff or appropriately loose. Pain and stiffness of the neck can occur with arthritis of the bones in the neck or in acute situations involving infections of the fluid around the brain (meningitis).

The doctor looks for abnormal fullness of the *jugular vein*, which is seen with backed up pressure in heart disease, and documents that the windpipe is in its normal midline location. The doctor may palpate (feel) the *thyroid* gland (the gland that controls the metabolic rate of the body), checking for abnormal masses or fullness. She will also check the lymph nodes in the neck. She may place the end of the stethoscope on either side of the neck on top of each *carotid artery*, listening for abnormal sounds suggestive of blood vessel narrowing or transmitted abnormal sounds from the heart, as in the case of heart murmurs.

Respiratory System

In examining the respiratory system, the doctor checks to see that chest expansion occurs equally on both sides and is not excessive (as occurs in emphysema), does not require accessory muscles to attain a breath, and that the chest cavity appears normal. The doctor taps (percusses) different parts of the chest, listening for hollow or dull sounds that help delineate normal air-filled lung from fluid-filled areas. With the use of the stethoscope, the doctor listens for abnormalities in breath sounds, such as wheezing or sounds of fluid in the chest. The respiratory exam is performed in both the sitting and lying positions, and in the front and the back parts of the chest.

The Breast

In the breast exam, the doctor methodically assesses any abnormal masses or discharge from the nipples, which can be signs of a tumor. The exam is performed in both the sitting and lying positions. Do not depend completely on your doctor's examination; ask him to show you how to properly examine your breasts for abnormalities. Of note, even men need to have their breasts examined for the rarer condition of breast cancer that occurs in men and for enlargement due to hormone imbalance.

The Heart

In examining the heart, the doctor uses the stethoscope to assess the heart rate, rhythm, and the two major component sounds of the heart beat. The doctor listens for abnormal sounds, such as extra beats and murmurs. Murmurs are the sound of blood flowing through abnormal valves or abnormal holes between chambers in the heart. (Valves are structures that are the gateways to different chambers of the heart or parts of major blood vessels.) The doctor also places a hand over the heart region of the chest to feel for abnormal thumping. The heart exam is performed in both the sitting and lying positions.

Limbs

In the examination of the limbs, the doctor checks for abnormal enlargement of the fingertips, abnormal discoloration of skin color, and swelling. Swelling is assessed by pressing a finger into the swollen area in order to see whether this leaves a temporary indentation or pitting. Swelling is a nonspecific sign of an abnormality in keeping the right amount of fluid within blood vessels and may be seen when the heart is not functioning properly due to backed up pressure, when protein levels are low in the bloodstream, or in kidney disease.

The fingertips and toes are examined for a progressive deformity that resembles the shape of a little club (*clubbing*) that may occur in conditions associated with low oxygen states, such as lung or heart disease, as well as liver and intestinal disorders, and in some types of cancer.

Vascular System

In the vascular exam, the normal throbbing from the arteries supplying the limbs (pulses) are checked and one side is compared to the other. A diminished pulse may be accompanied by reduced temperature of the limb.

The Spine

In examining the spine, the doctor looks for abnormal curvature, limitations of motion, or pain in reaction to mild pressure at different points. Tenderness at specific points along the spine may suggest a herniated disk or abnormal mass in that region.

The Abdomen (Belly)

In the abdominal exam, the stethoscope is used again to listen to the normal sounds produced by the intestines, called *bowel sounds*. Absent bowel sounds occur in late stages of intestinal obstruction, severe infections within the abdomen, or loss of blood flow to the intestine. Hyperactive bowel sounds occur in earlier phases of intestinal obstruction.

The doctor also listens for abnormal sounds from the large blood vessel running vertically through the abdomen known as the aorta. Enlargements or blockages of the aorta can be serious and may sometimes be detected by listening to these sounds. The doctor taps on the abdomen in order to outline the borders of the liver, located beneath the ribs on the person's right side, and the borders of the spleen, located below the ribs on the left. The doctor then proceeds to feel for the presence of abnormal masses and any enlargement of abdominal organs, such as the liver on the right or the spleen on the left. Abnormal bulging of a portion of the aorta can also be felt, indicating an abdominal aortic aneurysm. The doctor checks that the abdomen feels soft and that it is not expanded. For example, fluid swelling of the abdomen may be seen in severe liver disease. Areas that are tender to mild compression may suggest problems with the stomach, gallbladder, pancreas, or intestines. Involuntary, severe reflex muscle spasm in reaction to mild compression (guarding) may occur with serious infections within the abdomen.

Anal Region

In the rectal exam, the doctor checks for masses and feels for normal tone of the anal region known as the *sphincter*. The doctor may test a small sample of stool for the abnormal presence of blood. The rectal and stool exam are an important part of screening for malignancy. Be aware that stool samples may test falsely negative after a large intake of vitamin C, and they may test falsely positive due to eating meat in the few days preceding the exam. In a male, the doctor feels the prostate gland and assesses its size and texture.

Genitourinary Region

In the genitourinary exam of a man, the doctor examines the genitalia looking for lesions or discharge. The testicles are examined for abnormal tenderness or masses. In a woman, a formal pelvic exam includes a visual survey of the abdomen from the outer vaginal region, clitoris, and opening to the urinary tube (urethra). The internal examination uses a speculum to expose the mouth of the uterus (cervix). A Pap smear is performed to rule out cervical cancer, and a manual examination of the uterus and ovaries is performed by inserting one hand internally while pressing down with the other hand on the lower abdomen.

Musculoskeletal System

The musculoskeletal survey is an examination of the joints, bones, and muscles, during which the doctor notes any abnormal joint pain, tenderness, swelling, deformity, or diminished range of motion. The doctor also assesses any limitations of motion or soft tissue abnormalities.

Skin

During an examination of the skin, the doctor checks for the presence of lesions, ulcerations, or evidence of infection. Rashes can be a sign of a localized inflammation, a problem with an organ of the body, or reflect a widespread allergic reaction. Moles are inspected to insure they are not malignant (melanoma). Make sure that your doctor has allocated adequate time to examine your skin closely for this type of cancer.

Spots with specific patterns or coloring may suggest hereditary illnesses, such as neurofibromatosis. Pale skin suggests possible anemia, and bluish skin color suggests insufficient oxygen. Severely dry skin that stands up when pinched suggests dehydration. Sweaty skin in the absence of exertion can occur when the blood pressure drops. Blotches of bleeding spots suggest a bleeding tendency, such as a blood clot problem. The skin of people who are immobilized in bed should be examined for bed sores.

Lymph Nodes

Lymph nodes are collections of defense cells located throughout the body, especially in the neck, armpit, and groin areas. The doctor will check for abnormally enlarged lymph nodes, which are activated and tend to become enlarged when there is an infection, inflammatory illness, or a malignancy.

Neurologic Examination

The doctor begins the neurologic examination by assessing the level of consciousness and surveying the person's orientation and general thinking, language, and memory functions by asking a series of questions. Anything that affects the brain can cause changes in mental status. Examples are toxic effects (including prescribed or illegal drugs, alcohol), inflammation, infections, tumors, degenerative diseases of the brain cells or their connections, strokes or bleeding in the brain, changes in levels of elements in blood, such as sodium or glucose (sugar), head injury, and seizures. Changes in speech may be due to confusion, injuries to areas of the brain responsible for language function, or problems that affect the motor pronunciation of words.

The neurologic assessment is also known as the *mental status exam* and may include questions designed to identify psychiatric symptoms, such as paranoid thoughts, hallucinations, irrational thinking, depression, and anxiety.

The cranial nerves that come from the upper and lower parts of the brain affect primarily the movements and functions of parts of the face. They are tested sequentially by having the person perform numerous maneuvers. These include looking in different directions, lifting the eyebrows or making a smile, and sticking out the tongue, among others.

The motor portion of the neurologic exam is performed by asking the person to move different parts of the body against resistance offered by the doctor. The doctor also examines for abnormal movements of body parts, such as tremors, and assesses the resistance of body parts to being moved passively in what is called *tone*.

In the sensory exam, different modalities of sensation are tested, such as the ability to perceive light touch, pinprick, hot and cold, and movement of a body part in space. The doctor may tap a tuning fork and place it on a limb to test perception of vibration.

Tapping on joints throughout the body using a reflex hammer, the doctor checks for interruptions in the pathways from the limb to the brain and spinal cord, and then back to the limb again, which are demonstrated by a reduced reflex response, such as a reduced kick on one side when tapping the knee joint. Alternatively, exaggerated reflexes may suggest a brain or spinal cord problem. Increased or decreased reflexes also commonly occur in the absence of any problem. The heel of each foot may be stroked in order to observe whether the big toe abnormally elevates in a reflex known as the *Babinski response*, indicating an abnormality of nerve cells in the brain or spinal cord.

The doctor subsequently assesses coordination, which reflects the function of the hindbrain (cerebellum) and its many nerve connections. This is accomplished by having the person perform repetitive movements such as tapping of the finger or the foot, or having a finger reach for a target.

The final portion of the neurologic exam focuses on gait (walking). Since gait involves many of the neurologic functions—including thought, motor, sensory, and coordination—gait abnormalities can alert the doctor to diverse neurologic problems.

In summary, the physical examination provides the doctor with an opportunity to look for signs that contribute further information to the diagnostic process. Now that the history and all the squeezing and tapping have been completed, the doctor will select tests to further hone in on the diagnosis. We will learn all about the reasoning behind ordering tests in the next chapter.

CHAPTER 12

Testing Patients, Not Your Patience— Tests and Procedures

> "I was astounded when four technicians from four different depart-
> ments took four separate and substantial blood samples on the same
> day. That the hospital did not take the trouble to coordinate the tests,
> using one blood specimen, seemed to me inexplicable and irresponsi-
> ble. Taking four large slugs of blood the same day even from a healthy
> person is hardly to be recommended."

> NORMAN COUSINS
> *Anatomy of an Illness as Perceived by the Patient:*
> *Reflections on Healing and Regeneration*

Does your doctor go off on a wild goose chase, ordering test after test without any idea what your diagnosis may be? You might think that with the all
the advances in technology and the many tests available that the history and
examination offer very little in making a diagnosis. Indeed, some doctors hear
about a symptom and immediately order tests without any specific hypothe-
sis about what is going on. In our experience, this approach ends up creating
more confusion than clarification of the diagnosis. Only thoughtful, selective
use of tests and consideration before the test is ordered about how the results
will be used can lead to an accurate diagnosis.

Test information – Do not leave your doctor's office without it!

When your doctor hands you a prescription for a test, do you simply walk out
of his office without understanding what the test is for? Of course not; yet
people do this all the time, to varying degrees.

Your doctor should spend time explaining the procedure when he orders a
test. This discussion should include the risks and benefits, precautions,
preparations, and what to expect during the test, among other issues. You may
expect this information to be given automatically, but that does not necessarily happen. Be aggressive about obtaining this crucial information.

Form 10A provides questions that you can ask your doctor whenever a test
is ordered. Take this form with you to the doctor's office, fill it in yourself as
the doctor answers the questions, and keep it for future reference.

Getting answers to these questions will help you gain a better understanding of the nature, risks, and benefits of any testing procedure. In addition,

beyond these generic questions, there is a supplementary list of questions on Form 10B in the latter half of this chapter that is specific to the most common types of procedures.

Knowing the answers to these questions is not only important for your peace of mind. If the doctor neglects to tell you something about the test, it could also have serious medical repercussions. For example:

> Sixty-year-old Ms. Goldman wishes she had asked the right questions before going for a barium enema—a special kind of X-ray that can spot abnormalities in the large intestine. Good thing she mentioned to the X-ray technologist that she had breakfast earlier in the day so the test could be cancelled in time. It would have been nice if Dr. Goldman had warned her not to eat before the procedure, but it would *also* have been good if Ms. Goldman knew to ask.

> Mr. Squire had a similar problem. His doctor ordered an MRI (Magnetic Resonance Imaging) of his head. His doctor told him it was as simple as getting an X-ray. How could Mr. Squire have known in advance that he would get claustrophobic and feel like a hotdog that was being shoved into an enclosed donut! Too bad the test had to be cancelled. If the doctor had warned him about the common problem of claustrophobia during this test, or had Mr. Squire asked the right questions, he could have been sent to an open MRI facility or received something to calm him during the procedure.

My doctor ordered something called "ESR" when I told her about my joint pains. Will this test help her make a diagnosis?

Very few tests answer the basic question as to the presence or absence of a particular disease; most lend further evidence for or against a diagnosis in the same way that information in the history and physical exam do.[7] Tests are sometimes used not only to help generate a diagnosis, but rather to:

- Follow the course of an illness, such as clotting times of the blood (see below)

- Monitor treatment—for example, medical blood levels and assess risk factors for illness (lipid profile—see below)

7. *Diagnostic Tests: Smart Patient Good Medicine* by R.L. Sribnick and W.B. Sribnick. 1st? Ed. New York: Walker and Company, 1994:67-82.

- Monitor drug side effects, such as signs in the blood of allergic reactions to a medication

The next section describes some of the commonly used tests. If your doctor orders any of these tests, you can use the following discussion as reference.

Blood Tests

> My veins could sense her hesitation. Veins have their own peculiar survival technique in that they can actually retreat and hide. I do not know if it is a documented medical phenomenon, but I've seen it happen. Few things in this world are more ruthless than bad veins that can smell a phlebotomist's fear. As soon as the flat, falsetto tone of her voice reached my ears, I'd feel my veins constrict and shrink deeper under my skin. You could almost hear them chuckling.
>
> EVAN HANDLER
> *Time on Fire: My Comedy of Terrors*

The Complete Blood Count (CBC)

The CBC is one of the most common blood tests performed for screening purposes in healthy individuals. It is also used to monitor the health of individuals with medical disorders. One component of the CBC is the red blood cell. Red blood cells are responsible for transporting oxygen throughout the body; they contain an iron-containing substance called hemoglobin that binds to oxygen molecules. An increased red blood cell count (polycythemia) occurs as a normal reaction to compensate for decreased oxygen due to exposure to high altitudes. Alternatively it can be elevated in a disease state called *polycythemia vera*. Decreased numbers of red blood cells may occur when the generator of blood cells (the bone marrow) is not functioning properly, if blood is lost, or with abnormal destruction of the cells. The word *hematocrit* (Hct) is related to the RBC count and hemoglobin value and is a measure of the percentage of red blood cells in the volume of blood.

Red Blood Cells

The word *anemia* refers to an abnormally low number of red blood cells (decreased hemoglobin). The red blood cell count is near-normal in *iron deficiency anemia*, but each cell has an abnormally low content of hemoglobin. Such cells tend to have a paler color than usual (hypochromic) and tend to be smaller than normal (microcytic). Therefore, when investigating anemia, the doctor is also interested in indices that reflect the size of the cell (mean corpuscular volume) and hemoglobin content (mean corpuscular hemoglobin). However, people with an inherited disorder called *sickle cell* anemia have red blood cells that are normal in color and size. In anemia due to deficiencies of vitamin B12 or folic acid, the red blood cell is large. To further investigate anemia, the doctor may order blood tests related to iron, including iron levels (*ferritin*, the protein that stores iron) and the iron binding capacity, a measure of the ability of the protein in the blood (*transferrin*) to bind and transport iron.

Reticulocytes are immature cells that have not yet evolved into fully developed red blood cells. An increase in the number of reticulocytes may occur in response to the need for more red blood cells and indicates that the bone marrow is functioning and generating red blood cells. Alternatively, in certain forms of anemia, red blood cells are produced ineffectively and the reticulocyte count is low. Further investigation of anemia involves direct examination of blood cells under the microscope (smear) to observe their shape, which can help reveal the cause of the problem.

White Blood Cells

Another component of the CBC is the total white blood cell count. White blood cells are the defense cells of the body. The white blood cell count *differential* represents the percentage of different types of white blood cells, such as neutrophil, lymphocyte, monocyte, and eosinophil. During infections, the percentage of neutrophils increases and the relative percentage of lymphocytes decreases. An immature form of the neutrophil called a *band* also increases in numbers. Uncommon forms of bacterial infections and many viruses may cause a decrease in the neutrophil count. Individuals with very low neutrophil counts—for example, those undergoing chemotherapy—may be at particularly high risk for developing infections.

An increase in the eosinophil count is associated with allergic reactions or illness due to parasites. Lymphocytes may increase in response to viral infections or long-term bacterial infections. Acute or chronic lymphocytic leukemia is a malignancy associated with an increased lymphocyte count. A decrease in lymphocyte counts may be seen with some infections, such as human immunodeficiency virus (HIV). An increase in the monocyte count occurs in tuberculosis, in rare infections such as malaria, and very rarely in malignant conditions.

Electrolytes

Electrolytes are normally occurring chemicals in the blood and cells of the body. Sodium, potassium, and chloride are electrolytes that have varying concentrations inside and outside of our cells. They maintain the important electrical balance across the cell boundary necessary for cell function. Sodium tends to draw off water with it and, therefore, salt (sodium chloride) is restricted in the diets of individuals with heart disease or other conditions where fluids are abnormally retained in the body.

Increases in the sodium levels (hypernatremia) may be due to dehydration, excessive use of salt-containing fluids administered intravenously, or problems with kidney function. Low sodium levels (hyponatremia) may be due to excessive intake of fluids that do not contain salt, loss of sodium (from vomiting, diarrhea, or sweating), or from the effects of diuretics, which are medications that are used to stimulate the kidneys to eliminate fluid from the body but cause loss of sodium as well. Alternatively, problems with the kidneys or low levels of steroids can cause low sodium. (Steroids are naturally occurring chemicals in the body that are responsible for keeping sodium in the body, as well as having many other functions.)

The electrolyte *potassium* is needed for proper heart, nerve, and muscle function. An increase in potassium level (hyperkalemia) can be dangerous in the extreme, because it can lead to irregular heart rhythms and even arrested heartbeat. Potential causes of an increased potassium level include severe kidney disease, excessive potassium administered through an intravenous line, a temporary change after damage to a part of the body (muscle crush injury), or when there is high acidity in the bloodstream. Potassium levels can be falsely elevated if the fist is clenched during blood drawing.

Low levels of potassium may occur as a result of the use of diuretics (water pills), vomiting, or diarrhea, receiving steroid medications, or when the body is in a very low acid (alkalosis) state. Some water pills, such as aldactone, are called *potassium-sparing* and can increase potassium levels.

Calcium is obtained from the food we eat, and levels can be increased when parathyroid hormone—responsible for calcium balance in the body—is produced in excess, with malignancies, with the use of a type of diuretic called a *thiazide*, with severe inactivity, and with excessive intake of vitamin D. Calcium levels are falsely elevated when there is dehydration.

Low levels of calcium occur when an insufficient amount of parathyroid hormone is secreted, in kidney disease, with inflammation of the pancreas, and in severe malnutrition.

BUN and Creatinine

The *blood urea nitrogen* (BUN) test is a measure of the protein waste product *urea* that circulates in the blood on its way to the kidneys to be emptied from the body. Conditions that lead to increased breakdown of protein in the body, increased protein production—such as with gastrointestinal bleeding—very high-protein diets, or decreased circulating fluid volume in which the BUN is concentrated, can lead to an increased BUN. In the absence of these conditions, an elevated BUN indicates a problem with the kidneys.

Creatinine comes from muscle. It is a substance that is also excreted by the kidneys and can be used to estimate kidney function as well. The ratio of BUN to creatinine can give clues as to whether a kidney problem is related to dehydration or decreased blood flow to the kidneys, versus due to a problem of the kidneys themselves.

Glucose

Glucose is the natural sugar that the cells of our body use for energy. Insulin is a hormone secreted by the pancreas that drives glucose from the blood into the cells. In diabetes, there is problem with insulin production or resistance to the effects of insulin, which can lead to elevated blood sugars. When measuring the blood sugar (glucose) level, it is traditional to obtain a fasting level in order to screen for diabetes. Although it is advised not to eat anything for at least four hours before the test, water intake is permitted. Assessments for diabetes may include the *Glucose Tolerance Test* (GTT), which assesses how well the body returns blood sugar levels to normal after intake of a high dose of glucose. With prolonged elevation in blood sugar levels, the hemoglobin in red blood cells becomes bound with glucose. The hemoglobin A1C test is a measure of this sugar-hemoglobin complex that is sometimes used to see how well a person's diabetes is under control.

Diabetes is the most common cause of elevated blood sugar (hyperglycemia). Sugars also rise in response to steroids secreted from within the body or taken as a medication, from the adrenaline released in the body due to stress, or with abnormally high growth hormone secretion, such as in pituitary gland tumors.

A low blood sugar level (hypoglycemia) may occur due to abnormally low levels of the steroids secreted by the body, severe liver disease, or pituitary gland problems. Diabetics who administer too much insulin in relation to the amount of food ingested at any particular time may also get hypoglycemic. Most cases of low blood sugar are of unknown cause. In some cases, hypoglycemia occurs only reactively after having a meal.

Lipids (Fats)

Despite all the negative attention given to cholesterol, it is actually needed by the body for several reasons. It is even a component of the normal outer linings of all the cells in the body. Nevertheless, *too much* cholesterol is associated with developing plaques within blood vessels and the associated heart disease.

Why one person develops a high cholesterol level and others do not is not completely clear, but hereditary appears to play an important factor for some.

Triglycerides are another commonly measured fatty component in the blood. Genetic factors or disorders of the liver, kidney, pancreas, or thyroid can elevate triglyceride levels.

Fatty chemicals bound to proteins are called *lipoproteins* and are classified according to the density of the molecules. Low levels of high density lipoprotein cholesterol (HDL) are considered to be a risk factor for developing plaques within the vessels that supply the heart—a condition which is also known as coronary heart disease (CHD). Elevation of low-density lipoprotein cholesterol (LDL) and very low density lipoprotein (VLDL) are risk factors for CHD.

Prostate Specific Antigen

This blood test is a marker for benign or malignant growth of the prostate gland. It has provoked much controversy about its usefulness as a screening test for prostate cancer. It is very specific for prostate tissue abnormalities, but false-positive results have led to unnecessary interventions and it is unclear whether the early diagnosis of prostate cancer makes a difference in long-term outcome. However, many doctors rely on the results of this test to determine the necessity of further testing in their male patients.

Enzymes

The cells of our body contain chemicals called *enzymes*, which spill into the blood in greater than usual amounts when a part of the body is damaged. Most enzymes are found in different types of cells, and it may not be immediately clear which body part gave rise to an elevation in blood enzyme levels. Alkaline phosphatase is found in liver, bone, and other organs. In children, elevated alkaline phosphatase is normal and reflects the building of bone. In adults, increased alkaline phosphatase may be due to a medication that stimulates liver metabolism, or liver or gallbladder disease. Alternatively, problems with bone can increase this enzyme—for example, in Paget's disease and other bone-thickening conditions, or conditions where cancer has spread to bone. Abnormal elevation of liver enzymes can be a clue that the symptoms are caused by liver inflammation. Following the amount of liver enzyme elevation gives the doctor a clue whether the inflammation is worsening.

Acid phophatase is an enzyme produced by the prostate gland; it is tested as a marker for prostate cancer.

Other enzymes known as *transaminases* (SGOT and SGPT) are elevated after injury to the heart, such as during a heart attack, or with liver disease—

for example, viral hepatitis, medication-induced liver injury, alcohol-induced liver disease, and obesity-associated fatty liver.

Creatine kinase or creatine phosphokinase (CPK) is produced in skeletal muscle, heart muscle, and the brain. When the CPK level is elevated, a test for the subtypes of CPK (*isoenzymes*) may be ordered in order to clarify the source. Lactic dehydrogenase is an enzyme found in many organs that is also elevated with a heart attack, with red blood cell destruction, in acute damage to lung tissue, in some malignancies, with liver damage, severe drop in blood pressure, and with some forms of infection.

Amylase is an enzyme found in saliva and the pancreas that is often tested in the evaluation of abdominal pain to rule out pancreatitis.

Bilirubin

When red blood cells are old—approaching their usual four-month lifespan—and no longer functioning properly, they are broken down into a substance called unconjugated (indirect) *bilirubin*. Elevations in bilirubin levels may result in a yellow discoloration of the skin called *jaundice*. Some medical conditions, such as autoimmune diseases or sickle cell disease, are associated with the breakdown of red blood cells, and this may cause a rise in indirect bilirubin levels. In newborns, the immature red blood cells that remain are broken down, because the liver enzyme for modifying this indirect bilirubin is not fully developed until a few days after birth. This causes jaundice in newborns that tends to go away within a few days. Another cause for increase in indirect bilirubin in the newborn is when a blood factor known as *Rh* in the newborn is different than that of the mother, resulting in the latter producing antibodies that attack the Rh factor on the blood cells of the baby.

Indirect bilirubin is then sent to the liver to be modified in chemical structure (conjugated). Liver diseases in which the abnormality is that they are missing the chemical enzymes needed to alter the indirect bilirubin (Gilbert Syndrome) also result in elevated indirect bilirubin.

If the indirect bilirubin is modified successfully, its new form can be measured as conjugated (direct) bilirubin. Bilirubin is one of the components of bile stored in the gallbladder from where it is released into the intestines. If the duct from the gallbladder to the intestine that serves as a conduit for bile release is blocked (obstructed) by gallstones, a tumor, or other causes, the result is that increased direct bilirubin will be absorbed into the blood, causing *obstructive* jaundice. Sometimes, a distinct blockage cannot be identified, but some medications promote sluggishness of bile flow.

Therefore, in the presence of jaundice, the doctor order will order tests that can determine whether the bilirubin is direct or indirect. Other findings from the history, examination, and other tests of blood or liver function can give clues as to the origin of the jaundice.

C-Reactive Protein

C-reactive protein is a substance produced by the liver that can be measured in the bloodstream. Elevated levels signify that inflammation, infection or a cancerous growth is occurring somewhere in the body. It has also recently been demonstrated to be a marker for an elevated risk of heart attack or stroke.

Clotting Tests

The body's natural process to prevent bleeding is clotting, which involves 12 circulating protein factors, each of which can be disrupted in different ways. The medication warfarin (Coumadin®) affects one of these clotting factors and the degree to which it does so can be measured as the prothrombin time (PT) or international normalized ratio (INR). Following these clotting times guides fine adjustments to the dosage of warfarin. People receiving warfarin should check with the doctor about foods and medications that can interfere with the effects of the medication. In the absence of warfarin as a cause for increased PT, other causes include liver disease and gastrointestinal disorders that prevent the absorption of vitamin K, which is needed to make some of the clotting factors. Elevated partial thromboplastin time (PTT) occurs with the use of an intravenous blood thinner, such as heparin, in bleeding disorders due to the absence of a clotting factor, or as a reaction to a severe generalized body illness.

Platelets are fragments of blood cells that are usually measured as part of the CBC. As platelets come together, they release chemicals that begin the clotting process. Abnormally increased platelet counts may occur with malignancies, accompanying an abnormally high red blood cell count in the disease polycythemia vera, or after the spleen is removed—elimination of the spleen means a loss of the blood cell breakdown normally performed by the spleen.

Low platelet count (thrombocytopenia) can be of unknown cause, part of an autoimmune or viral illness, or resulting from diseases or interventions that affect the bone marrow—for example, in people receiving chemotherapy. (As previously stated, red blood cells are produced by the bone marrow.) Platelet counts can also be lowered by diseases or medications that lead to the destruction of platelets. If platelet counts become extremely low, the risk of bleeding is greatly increased.

Hormones

The glands in the body produce hormones that have specific functions in different parts of the body. Some hormones are produced by the pituitary gland

and brain; others are released from the adrenal glands, parathyroid and thyroid gland, the pancreas, the testes, and the ovaries. Based on symptoms or signs on physical examination, the doctor may be suspicious of an abnormally low or high production of a hormone. Blood tests to measure hormone levels include the following: pituitary hormone level [which includes growth hormone (GH)], adrenocorticotropin (ACTH), thyroid stimulating hormone (TSH), follicle-stimulating hormone (FSH), luteinizing hormone (LH), and prolactin. Hormones produced by the adrenal glands can be measured as cortisol levels, aldosterone levels, vanillylmandelic acid (VMA), or metanephrines. Parathyroid hormone levels can also be assessed. Thyroid function tests include: free T4 index, T-3 and T-4 levels, and TSH. Testosterone, estrogen, and progesterone levels reflect hormones secreted by the testes and ovaries.

Drug Levels

When a medication is prescribed, there may be reasons to measure its level in the bloodstream, including: [8]

1. Assessing whether the dose given is achieving a therapeutic range. This range is determined by assessing a large number of individuals and seeing which levels are associated with the drug achieving its desired effect without causing side effects in most people. The problem is that what is good for the majority of people may not necessarily be good for a specific individual; some people need high levels of medication and some do very well with low levels. Doctors should place priority on how a person is doing clinically rather than focusing completely on blood tests.

2. When a person cannot express to the doctor whether they are having dose-related side effects, because levels are a rough guide to the likelihood of drug toxicity.

3. To assess whether a person is actually taking the drug as instructed.

4. When there is liver or kidney disease, which may disrupt the normally expected levels and lead to the need to alter the usual drug dosage.

5. When different types of drugs are being mixed, giving rise to the risk for drug interactions. Among the different types of drug interactions are those that overstimulate the liver to metabolize the second drug, resulting in a lower level of the latter drug. Alternatively, the first drug may inhibit the liver from metabolizing the second drug, resulting in

8. *Diagnostic Tests: Smart Patient Good Medicine* by R.L. Sribnick and W.B. Sribnick. 1st Ed. New York: Walker and Company, 1994:67-82.

an abnormally elevated level of the second drug. Drugs may compete with each other for space on the proteins that transport the drugs to different parts of the body.

When more than one drug is administered and it is unclear which drug is mainly responsible for the problem, the drug associated with the elevated level may be responsible.

6. To determine if an illegal drug is being used.

7. When an individual arrives at an emergency room after having swallowed or injected an unknown substance.

8. When an individual has overdosed on a medication.

Examples of drugs whose levels may be monitored routinely include certain antibiotics, antiepileptic drugs, medications used for severe psychiatric conditions, antiasthma drugs, digoxin (a heart drug), and drugs used to control heart rhythms.

Urinalysis

Analysis of the components of urine can provide many clues to disorders of the kidneys and other organs of the body. The color of urine may be changed by many types of medications due to the presence of blood or with certain types of infection. The pH of the urine indicates the amount of acidity. Low acidity (increased alkalinity) can promote the formation of certain types of kidney stones and infections. Specific gravity, which measures the concentration of components in the urine, is increased when an individual is dehydrated, has a hormonal problem that leads to insufficient emptying of fluids, or contains an excess of sugars or proteins. Decreased specific gravity occurs after drinking a very large volume of fluid, in some cases dangerously excessive.

The urinalysis also detects the abnormal presence of proteins in the urine, which may indicate leakage of proteins from diseased kidneys or spilling of proteins excessively produced in the body due to malignancy. High blood pressure and diabetes may also be associated with protein in the urine.

Sugar in the urine occurs in diabetes. A high number of red blood cells in the urine suggests bleeding in the urinary tract system, but contamination of the urine sample by menstrual blood flow should be excluded. A significant number of white blood cells in the urine suggests infection or inflammation. Clumping of proteins and cells called *casts* found in the urine suggests kidney disease. Bacteria in small numbers in the urine usually suggests contamination from regions around the urinary outlet. Significant numbers of bacteria accompanied by high urinary white blood cell counts suggest infection. A positive test for leukocyte esterase in the urine further supports the diagnosis of an infection. A urinary bacterial culture is performed when infection is suspected. The microbiology laboratory will also assess the sensitivity of the bacteria and its vulnerability to being killed by different antibiotics.

Less commonly, an entire 24-hour collection of urine is obtained to look for chemical evidence of unusual diseases, such as porphyria or rare tumors of the gastrointestinal tract (carcinoid tumors). People undergoing such testing should ask the doctor which foods or drugs should be avoided before the test so there is no interference with test results.

FORM 10A

Test and Procedure Questions

What is the test called? _____

Where will the test be performed? Will it require hospitalization? _____

_____

What is the purpose of the test? _____

_____

What are the risks associated with the test? How common are the risks? ____

_____

Are there any alternatives to having the test? _____

How much experience has the person doing this examination had with this test? _____

_____

Have they had any complications in doing it? _____

Are there any special preparations, precautions, or eating or activity restrictions before the test? _____

_____

Is there any special clothing that should be worn? _____

How does the test work? How is the test performed? _____

_____

What will the patient do during the test? _____

Does the test involve receiving any medications or intravenous insertion? ___

_____

How will the test feel? Is it uncomfortable? _____

How long does it take? _____

What happens after the test? _____

Are there any special instructions, precautions, or activity restrictions to follow after the test? _____

_____

What symptoms should I be concerned about after the test? What symptoms should the doctor be notified about? Which symptoms can be ignored?

_____

_____

What should be done if a complication from the test develops? _____

_____

How and when can I obtain test results? _____

When should a follow-up appointment be made? _____

_____

Will further tests be necessary after this test? _____

Will insurance cover the cost of the test? _____

Questions to Ask About Specific Tests

If your doctor orders specific tests, you may want to ask him questions such as the following. Take the portion of this form that applies to you (and the test your doctor has ordered) with you to the doctor's office, fill it in yourself as the doctor answers the questions, and keep it for future reference.

Arteriogram (Cerebral)

This procedure involves injection of a dye through a catheter (tube) that is inserted into a blood vessel in the groin. It is used to identify and characterize areas of narrowing in blood vessels supplying the brain.

Questions to ask your doctor:

How experienced is the doctor performing this procedure? _____

_____

What are the risks, including the possibility of loosening an existing blood clot or puncturing a major blood vessel? What is the risk of a stroke? _____

_____

_____

What emergency precautions are in place, should a serious complication develop? _____

_____

Is my kidney function good enough to handle the dye that will be injected?

_____

Barium Enema

A barium enema is an X-ray of the lower gastrointestinal tract, which is outlined by administering the contrast material barium through the rectum. This test helps identify structural abnormalities, such as cancers or inflammation of the lower gastrointestinal tract.

Questions to ask your doctor:

What are the risks of the barium passing through the wall of the intestine?

_____

_____

Do I have any conditions that make the barium enema risky to perform? ___

_____

Biopsy of Skin

Skin biopsy involves the sample of a small amount of skin tissue under local numbing medication in order to determine the pathology of a skin abnormality and to rule out a malignancy.

Questions to ask your doctor:

What medications can I take if the biopsy site is painful after the procedure? _____

_____

How do I take care of the biopsy site? _____

_____

When are the sutures removed and when should I be seen for a follow-up?

_____

Biopsy of Bone Marrow

Bone marrow aspiration and biopsy involves taking a sample of the inner core of a bone in order to gain information about blood disorders, such as anemia or blood cell line malignancies. It involves inserting a needle under local anesthesia, usually into a bone in the back of the pelvis.

Questions to ask your doctor:

What should I look for to rule out bleeding, infection, or inflammation at the biopsy site? _____

_____

How will the results of the test change the plan of treatment? _____

_____

_____

Computed Axial Tomography (CAT) Scan

This picture of a body part can identify structures poorly seen on X-ray and provide much more detail. It involves lying flat on a table and entering a machine that is shaped like a donut.

Questions to ask your doctor:

If a material called a *contrast agent* is to be injected intravenously during the procedure, are there any risk factors for an increased tendency toward allergic reactions to the contrast agent? _____

_____

What are the risks associated with the dye—for example, allergic reactions or kidney problems? _____

_____

What can be done if I experience claustrophobia (fear of enclosed spaces)?

_____

Are there any risks associated with being exposed to radiation? _____

Catheterization of the Heart

This procedure involves the insertion of catheters (tubes) through the blood vessels into the heart in order to reveal the outline of the heart and the blood vessels supplying it. Catheterization is used mainly to identify and characterize areas of narrowing in the blood vessels.

Questions to ask your doctor:

How experienced is the doctor in performing this procedure? _____

_____

What are the risks, including the possibility of loosening an existing blood clot or developing a heart attack or a stroke? _____

_____

What emergency precautions are in place, should a serious complication develop? _____

_____

Is my kidney function good enough to handle the dye that will be injected?

_____

Echocardiography

This test uses ultrasound waves to obtain images of the heart. It can be helpful in assessing abnormal thickening of heart muscle, abnormally increased or decreased size of heart chambers, abnormalities in the valves that separate the chambers of the heart, and how well the heart is pumping blood.

Questions to ask your doctor:

Will I need to swallow the probe [Transesophageal Echocardiogram (TEE)]?

_____

_____

If so, what are the associated risks? _____

_____

Electroencephalography (EEG)

The EEG is a test that measures the electrical waves generated by the brain. It involves the application of little metal cups to the scalp using paste. These cups are then connected to an EEG machine by wires. The EEG is useful in looking for signs of change in brain function, such as changes caused by medications or dementing illnesses, including Alzheimer's disease. It is also crucial in the evaluation of seizures.

Should I take my regular medications on the day of the test? _____

Should I stay up the night before the test? (Sleep deprivation is sometimes used to promote sleeping during the test in order to bring out certain abnormalities.) _____

_____

How is the EEG paste best removed at home, after the test is over? _____

_____

Electromyography (EMG) and Nerve Conduction Velocity Testing

These two tests measure the health of the nerve pathways outside the brain and the muscles they supply. EMG involves the insertion of a fine needle into selected muscles to assess abnormalities in the normal electrical signal produced in the muscle. Nerve conduction testing involves giving a small electrical signal along one part of the nerve and measuring how quickly it is received at another point along the nerve.

Notify your doctor before an EMG is done if you are taking blood thinners because they can raise the risk of bleeding from the test. _____

_____

Endoscopy (Upper Endoscopy or Colonoscopy)

Endoscopy involves the use of a scope device to peer into the inside of a hollow part of the body, such as the stomach, the large intestine (colon), or throat. Endoscopy of the upper gastrointestinal tract involves insertion of a fiber optic device, while under sedation, down the esophagus and into the stomach and the first part of the small intestine. This test looks for inflammation, tumors, and ulcers, and permits biopsies of any abnormalities found.

Colonoscopy involves insertion of the colonoscope through the rectum into the large intestine in order to assess inflammatory diseases, determine the source of gastrointestinal bleeding, and identify structural abnormalities, such as polyps or tumors.

Questions to ask your doctor:

What are the risks of puncturing any of the structures the scope is inserted into? _____

_____

What signs should I notify the doctor about after I return home from the procedure? _____

_____

What kind of bowel preparation will be needed? Will it cause cramps and diarrhea? _____

_____

Exercise Stress Test

This test provides clues as to the adequacy of blood flow to the heart by having an individual walk on a treadmill or ride a stationery bicycle in order to place stress on the heart. This can bring out abnormal patterns on the electrocardiogram due to insufficient blood flow and oxygen—resulting from the increased demands on the heart—and indicate whether the heart is not getting enough circulation. Stress tests may be supplemented with the use of a radioisotope, such as thallium, a substance that helps outline the areas of heart that are receiving inadequate blood supply.

Questions to ask your doctor:

Will the test be done using the radioisotope? _____

How will the test be performed if I cannot do the exercise? _____

_____

Is there a possibility I will develop chest pain or even have a heart attack while doing this test? _____

_____

Intravenous Pyelography (IVP)

This is an X-ray of the kidneys and its connections (ureters and bladder) that is performed with the use of a dye. It can show abnormalities in the structure of the urinary tract and identify stones.

Questions to ask your doctor:

Discuss any history of asthma or prior allergic reactions to iodine-containing substances. Is an anti-inflammatory drug (steroids) needed? _____

_____

Is my kidney function healthy enough to undergo this test? _____

How much fluid should I drink after the procedure and for how long? _____

_____

Lumbar Puncture (Spinal Tap and Cerebrospinal Fluid Analysis)

The lumbar puncture (LP) is a sampling of fluid that surrounds the brain and spinal cord. With the use of local numbing medication, a thin needle is inserted into the lower spine area in a region where the nerve roots are bathed in cerebrospinal fluid (CSF). Analysis of the CSF is then performed to measure pressure and look for evidence of infection, inflammation, bleeding, and malignancy.

Questions to ask your doctor:

Is the doctor sure there is no abnormal mass in the brain that could cause brain compression as a reaction to changes in fluid pressure caused by the LP? _____

_____

What side effects can be expected from the procedure? What will be done if headaches develop? _____

_____

Is an experienced doctor performing the test? _____

How long do I have to lie flat after the procedure? _____

Magnetic Resonance Imaging (MRI)

This test can take a very fine picture of the inner structures of any body part, such as the brain, and it is generally superior to a computed axial tomography scan (CAT). It involves lying flat on a table and going into a partially enclosed chamber.

Questions to ask your doctor:

Was any metal implanted in my body during a prior surgical procedure? (Since the MRI uses magnetic fields to produce pictures, there are safety risks if you have a cardiac pacemaker or other metal is implanted in your body.) _____

_____

What can be done if I experience claustrophobia (fear of enclosed spaces)?

_____

Mammogram

This X-ray of the breasts is used as a screening procedure to look for early evidence of growths. There are many controversies surrounding both its usefulness in detecting early-stage breast cancer and how often it should be performed.

Questions to ask your doctor:

How often does the doctor want a mammography to be performed? _____

_____

Will it be done at the best available radiology center with qualified radiologists interpreting the films? _____

_____

Remind your doctor if you have breast implants, because mammograms involve compression of the breasts between two film plates. _____

_____

Nuclear Scans

Nuclear (radionuclide) scans are pictures of parts of the body, such as bone, lung, liver, thyroid, and brain that can show changes in structure as well as aspects of function. These scans are often helpful in detecting areas of inflammation, such as from poorly identified fractures, infections, or tumors. The procedure involves the use of small amounts of radioactive substances, although the radiation risk tends to be in the same range as routine X-rays.

Questions to ask your doctor:

Are there any specific risks due to the radiation used in the procedure? _____

_____

If you are breastfeeding or there is any possibility you are pregnant, tell your doctor before any testing is done. _____

Ophthalmoscopy

This test involves using an ophthalmoscope to look at the back of the eye (the retina) where observed blood vessels, the end of the nerve involved in vision, and the spot where images are focused is located. Abnormalities can be clues to diverse problems, including high blood pressure, bleeding in the brain, clots coming from the heart, complications of diabetes, and increased pressure in the brain. Eye drops may be used in order to dilate the pupils.

Will my eyesight be blurry after the procedure? _____

Will I be able to drive home? _____

Papanicolaou (Pap) Smear

The Pap smear is a procedure to collect some of the cells that are sloughed off the walls of the outside portion of the uterus known as the cervix to check for signs of malignancy. They are analyzed for their *cytology* (cellular characteristics) and then classified as appearing normal, atypical but with no evidence of malignancy, or showing varying degrees of malignancy. Sometimes the word *dysplasia* is used to describe premalignant cells.

Questions to ask your doctor:

Clarify whether the Pap test can be done when you are menstruating. _____

_____

Discuss with the doctor whether intercourse or douching should be avoided for 48 hours before the Pap smear is performed. _____

_____

If the Pap smear is abnormal, how serious are the findings and what further testing needs to be done? _____

_____

Pulmonary Function Tests

These tests measure the quality of breathing function. They are useful to determine the severity of lung diseases, such as bronchitis or emphysema. The test involves blowing in and out of tubes connected to devices that measure the force of breathing.

Questions to ask your doctor:

Are there any preparations before the test? _____

_____

Can I resume my normal activities after the test is done? _____

In the next chapter, we will learn how the doctor puts all the information together and arrives at a diagnosis.

CHAPTER 13

Putting it all Together – How the Doctor Arrives at the Diagnosis

> "One of my first reactions when lupus was finally diagnosed was; 'Oh, thank God! I'm not crazy!' Because having strange symptoms for so long a time, you wonder if they're imaginary. And lupus has so many fuzzy things about it. It is not like having heart disease or something like that where you know that that is what's giving out on you."
>
> CHERI REGISTER
> *Living with Chronic Illness: Days of Patience and Passion*

In the preceding chapters, we examined the medical evaluation in piecemeal fashion. In this section, we provide an illustrative emergency room case in order to demonstrate how the doctor puts the components of the medical evaluation together and arrives at a *differential diagnosis*. Mrs. Thorn, described below, has been prudently maintaining detailed records about her medical history and is able to provide them to the emergency room doctor, greatly assisting in his ability to accurately diagnose and treat her acute condition. This case demonstrates the importance of having your history available *before* an emergency occurs. (A copy of Mrs. Thorn's personal records can be found in Appendix A on page 231.)

Emergency Room Case Records of Mrs. Thorn
Chief Complaint (See Chapter 1)

Mrs. Thorn is a 60-year-old woman who arrives at the emergency room with a chief complaint of new-onset headaches over the past seven hours.

Comment:

Believe it or not, with as little as a one sentence chief complaint, the astute doctor can generate a differential diagnosis. Doctors who think in these terms before plunging into the history, exam, and testing are more likely to arrive at a diagnosis than those who mindlessly seek information in a rote fashion.

The doctor considers a number of broad categories, such as tumors, infections, migraines, medications, metabolic causes, tension headaches, high blood pressure, musculoskeletal problems in the neck, eye strain, glaucoma, strokes, and hemorrhages, among others. Even without taking a further history, this list can be narrowed by knowledge about the typical presentation of each diagnosis.

For example, the doctor knows that it is unusual to develop migraines at age 60, and tumors that cause high blood pressure are rare (particularly at Mrs. Thorn's age). Further reduction of this broad list of possibilities is achieved by proceeding with the History of Present Illness, which elicits information that either supports or discourages each diagnosis.

History of Present Illness (See Chapter 2)

Mrs. Thorn was in her usual good state of health until seven hours earlier, and although she has experienced occasional headaches in the past, they were nothing like her current symptoms. This headache began suddenly while she was sitting in a chair watching television. It felt like an explosion, starting and remaining all over her head, but worst towards the back of her head. It began and continues to be an excruciating, intense, continuous feeling of pressure. On a scale of 1 to 10, where 10 is the worst, she rates the headache as a 9. She describes it as the "worst headache of my life."

There was no obvious precipitant for Mrs. Thorn's headache. For example, she did not recently begin any new medications. The headache remained unchanged in severity after taking two acetaminophen tablets. She lay down but was unable to fall asleep. She began to feel nauseous near the time the headache started, which has persisted. She vomited once. She also feels that her left hand is not able to grip properly. The weakness developed one hour after the headache began. Her husband also had the impression that she does not have full use of her left hand. Currently, she feels quite anxious that something catastrophic has occurred in her head.

Past Medical History (See Chapter 4)

Past medical history is notable for tonsillectomy at age seven and removal of appendix at age 13. She was evaluated at age 50 for lower back pain that was diagnosed as arthritis and resolved near the time it began. There is no history of high blood pressure or any neurologic diseases.

Family History (See Chapter 5)

Mrs. Thorn and her husband have no children. Her mother died from a stroke at the age of 72, and her father died at age 70 from complications of diabetes mellitus. She has one sister, age 55, who is healthy.

Prior Diagnostic Workup (See Chapter 6)

Mrs. Thorn's prior diagnostic workup consisted of X-rays of the lower back, which were performed ten years earlier and showed mild arthritic changes.

Current and Prior Treatments (See Chapter 7)

Mrs. Thorn currently takes no medications. Prior medications consisted of ibuprofen and acetaminophen, which were taken ten years earlier for her lower back pain.

Psychosocial History (See Chapter 8)

Mrs. Thorn lives with her husband, who is in good health. She describes herself as "happily married." They have no children. Mrs. Thorn has worked in a high stress position as an accountant in a major airplane manufacturer. Her husband is an executive in an investment firm.

Review of Systems (See Chapter 10)

Overall is unremarkable.

Physical Examination (See Chapter 11)

She appeared to be in moderate distress because of pain. Vital signs included elevated blood pressure of 170/88 and pulse of 89; temperature was normal at 98^5 and respirations were normal at 12 per minute.

Head and neck examination was notable for rigidity of neck flexion. The remainder of the general physical examination was normal. On neurologic examination, she was alert and her thinking and language function were intact. Motor testing revealed weakness of the muscles in the left hand, and she was slightly weak extending her left arm at the elbow. She was also slightly weak flexing the left leg at the hip.

Comment:

Let us review the doctor's original list of possibilities and see how information from the history and examination support or discourage each diagnosis. This list included: tumors, infections, migraines, medications, metabolic causes, tension headaches, high blood pressure, musculoskeletal problems in the neck, eye strain, glaucoma, strokes, and hemorrhages.

A tumor in the brain is possible, but a more classic history would be of a progressive, more prolonged course of headaches. Infections such as encephalitis (infection of the brain) or meningitis (infections in the fluid-filled lining of the brain and spinal cord) are possibilities but they tend to have more a gradual onset, more prolonged duration, and are often associated with fever.

It is unusual for migraine headaches to develop for the first time at this age, and this form of presentation is unusual. She is on no medications that could cause headaches, and the headache is unusually severe for a tension headache. She has no history of high blood pressure. Other causes, such as dental disease and eye strain, are very unlikely to cause this type of severe, unremitting headache and would not be expected to cause a neurologic problem, such as limb weakness.

Headaches that begin suddenly with no prior history of significant headaches are worrisome because they may indicate an acute, serious event in the head, such as *ischemic* stroke (brain injury due to sudden lack of blood flow to a part of the brain) or hemorrhage (bleeding). One particularly classic form of bleeding (*subarachnoid hemorrhage*) is notoriously associated with a sudden, excruciating, and persistent headache. Neck rigidity further supports the possibility of bleeding (which is suggestive of irritation of the lining of the brain, as may occur with bleeding), nausea, and vomiting. Brain injury due to insufficient blood flow or hemorrhage may be associated with the neurologic abnormalities seen on Mrs. Thorn's examination.

Tests:

The next phase of the evaluation is designed to confirm suspected diagnoses by ordering appropriate tests. Routine blood work, such as blood counts, will be helpful in looking for low platelet counts that could lead to bleeding, anemia that could cause headaches, clotting factors, and metabolic abnormalities (see Chapter 12).

Because the doctor is concerned about possible hemorrhage or stroke, an emergency CAT scan of Mrs. Thorn's head is ordered (see Form 10B for a description of CAT scans, page 90).

As suspected, this test reveals extensive amounts of bleeding in the brain. Further testing reveals the presence of a bulging blood vessel known as an *aneurysm*, which has ruptured. Surgery is performed and thankfully Mrs. Thorn enjoys an uncomplicated recovery.

Final thoughts:

While this hypothetical case presents an idealized version of thorough history-taking and prompt evaluation, less organized and less detailed information could have resulted in the failure to recognize a very serious diagnosis. While the burden is on the doctor to consider the broad differential diagnosis, providing a detailed history greatly assists the doctor in formulating important possibilities and acting on them.

CHAPTER 14

To Waste Time or Not Waste Time, That Is the Question—The Follow-up Visit and Specific Diagnoses

"'The source of the tumor is your right testicle,' Dr. Klein explained. He said the tumor formed from the drainage of cancerous cells through my lymph, starting from my testicular region. In the ultrasound, they had found some scar tissue on my right testicle and told me they were 100 percent sure that was what caused the tumor, even though I did not have a prominent lump. In some men, the symptoms can cause enormous swelling in that region, but not in my case.

After the doctors gave their diagnosis, dead air filled the office. I looked around at all the somber faces and decided to break the ice.

'Oh, is that all?' I deadpanned. 'I thought it was going to be something serious.'… But my doctors did not react, not even a smirk."

SCOTT HAMILTON
Landing It: My Life On and Off the Ice

When I returned to see the doctor for a second visit, I dwelled on my back pain problem. I completely forgot to ask him questions about the irregular heart beat he had diagnosed the last time I saw him.

As important as it is to prepare for the initial visit with the doctor, it is equally important to organize information for follow-up visits. On the initial visit, you and the doctor faced the daunting challenge of integrating a vast quantity of information. On the follow-up visit, you and your doctor need to quickly piece together your history from the conclusions of the last encounter, analyze test results, and see how well your symptoms responded to treatments. It will be easy for both of you to get lost in a quagmire of information if you suffer from multiple medical problems. To make matters worse, follow-up visits are usually allotted much less time than the initial visit. When you are with the doctor and the waiting room is teeming with people looking at their watches, you may not feel like you have the time you need to cover everything.

How to Optimize Time with the Doctor

The solution is to organize your medical information and questions before you go to the doctor's office. By preparing symptom and medication-related information ahead of time, you will be able to free up more time for discussion with the doctor and avoid wasting time trying to recall details. On the other hand, even with the most efficient advance preparation of information, the issue to be discussed may require more time than that typically allotted for in a follow-up office visit. In that case, you and your doctor need to discuss either extending the duration of the appointment or consider returning for another appointment to continue the discussion.

Form 11 will help you prepare for your follow-up visit.

First and foremost, remind your doctor when your last encounter was. For example, if you were not seen for several years, the doctor may need to start over with a new comprehensive evaluation. If your last evaluation was one week ago, the office visit will likely be more focused on a specific issue. If the last encounter was a phone conversation, you can cite the nature of what was discussed.

Now you should provide details about each of your active medical problems. Referring to your problem list, describe step-by-step what happened during any episodes that have occurred since the last visit. If there were no repeat episodes, indicate it. If you have a chronic persistent problem simply describe how it feels recently. For each description, include the following information:

- Anything that tends to bring on an episode
- Anything that makes it worse
- What you were doing when it came on
- Any warning feelings that an episode is about to occur
- Where you were when the episode occurred
- The time the episode occurred
- What was done in response to having an episode
- Anything that made your symptoms get better, or anything that did not work
- Any associated symptoms
- A step-by-step description of what you experienced during the episode
- What others observed during the episode
- How long the episode lasted
- What symptoms were experienced after the episode was over

For example, a 60-year-old woman who has been followed for the problems of heartburn and back pain lists each problem separately, noting the dates of each attack and describing it:

1. Name of problem: Heartburn

Date of episode: 2/15/02

Description:

I suddenly woke up from sleep at 2 A.M. with a mild burning feeling in the upper part of my belly that rose up to my throat. I was burping frequently at the beginning of the attack. I was also nauseous for several minutes during the episode. The whole episode lasted for five minutes and was relieved by taking an antacid.

Date of episode: 3/14/02

Description:

One hour after a breakfast consisting of granola cereal and coffee, I experienced a typical burning feeling in my upper belly that rose to my chest. It was immediately relieved by taking an antacid tablet.

2. Name of Problem: Back Pain

Date of episode: 2/17/02

Description:

After sitting in a chair at the computer for two hours, I experienced a worsening of my usual lower back pain. It was a dull ache in the lower back that became sharp when I bent over. It lasted for two days. It did not seem to get better when I took the ibuprofen that was prescribed.

Date of episode: 4/18/02

Description:

After jogging around a track for one hour, I began to experience a sharp pain in my lower back that traveled down the back of my right leg to the ankle area. The pain was mild and lasted for about three hours. I tried lying down flat with my knees slightly bent and this seemed to help relieve the pain.

Highlighting Symptoms of Specific Diagnoses

If your diagnosis has been established, your doctor will have specific questions relevant to your particular diagnosis. Here is a list of some of the most common medical conditions and associated symptoms, which can be used to prepare you for the questions you can expect when you see the doctor.

Arthritis: Joint inflammation. Describe any stiffness, pain or swelling in joints, visual changes, chest pains, shortness of breath, and lack of energy.

Asthma: Inflammation and narrowing of the breathing airways. Describe any shortness of breath, wheezing, cough, or symptoms of a cold.

Brain Disorders: This category includes any brain mass, such as a tumor, infection, blood clot, or stroke, or other neurologic diagnoses, such as head trauma or multiple sclerosis. Note headaches, change in ability to think or speak, change in behavior, dizziness, nausea or vomiting, blurring or loss of vision, difficulty swallowing, weakness or numbness in the face or rest of the body, coordination problem, seizures, or loss of control over bowel or bladder function.

Bronchitis (inflammation of the lungs) or Pneumonia: Tell the doctor about any cough, including whether it is productive of phlegm, the color of the phlegm, wheezing, shortness of breath, fatigue, fever, or pain in the chest when taking a deep breath.

Cancer of Blood Cells (Leukemia) or Lymph Glands (Lymphoma): Explain any fatigue, fever, colds or other infections, swollen lymph glands, tendency to bruise easily, nose bleeds, aching joints, weight loss, change in appetite, feeling of fullness in the abdomen, or night sweats.

Chronic Fatigue Syndrome: A poorly-understood medical problem consisting of debilitating exhaustion and very low stamina lasting over six months. The cause remains unknown. Describe other symptoms, such as memory and concentration difficulties, headaches, swollen tender lymph nodes, sore throat, muscle aches, joint pains, or unrefreshing sleep.

Colon Cancer: Note any changes in bowel habits, new problems with constipation or diarrhea, abdominal pain, blood in the stool, or weight loss.

Coronary Artery Disease (Angina and Heart Attack): Indicate any symptoms of heart failure (see "Heart Failure" entry in this list), chest pain, palpitations, or shortness of breath. Since stroke may be a complication of heart disease, mention any symptoms that may suggest this (see entry "Mass in Brain" in this list).

Deep Vein Thrombosis: This is a condition where a blood clot forms in the large veins of the legs, which carries the risk of breaking off and traveling into the blood vessels supplying the lungs (pulmonary embolus). Describe any symptoms of swelling and pain in your legs.

Diabetes Mellitus: A condition associated with lack of production of insulin (a hormone that drives sugar into cells) or abnormalities in the response of the cells to insulin. Note the frequency of urination, degree of thirst, hunger, lack of energy, chest pains, shortness of breath, new problems with weakness or numbness, changes in vision, infections on the skin or established skin sores, sexual difficulties, wounds that do not heal well, numbness or stinging pains in the limbs, constipation or diarrhea, loss of control over bowel and bladder, problems with vision, lightheadedness, or breaking into a sweat.

Fibromyalgia Syndrome: A poorly understood disorder of pain and tenderness in the soft tissues surrounding bones, muscles, and joints. Describe where you are experiencing pain and how the pain is affected by activity, the weather, and stress. Note possible associated symptoms, such as fatigue, difficulty concentrating, disrupted sleep, headaches, anxiety, gastrointestinal symptoms, or a sensation of swelling in painful areas.

Gallbladder Disease (gallstones): Describe any abdominal pain, yellowing of skin, change in appetite, fever, or clay-colored stools.

Gastroesophageal Reflux Disease (GERD): A condition associated with the backup of stomach contents into the esophagus, or hiatal hernia, in which part of the stomach is abnormally squeezed into the chest area. Highlight any symptoms of heartburn, persistent cough, or abnormal sensation in the throat.

Hay Fever: Describe stuffy nose, runny nose, nasal congestion, sneezing, sore throat, and eyes that are itchy, irritated, tearing, or red.

Heart Failure: This is a condition in which the heart does not pump blood effectively to the rest of the body. Tell the doctor about any shortness of breath —including when lying flat or on exertion, and how many pillows are needed for sleeping—lack of energy, cough (including coughing up fluid or blood), palpitations, swelling in the legs, swelling of the abdomen, losing or gaining weight, lightheadedness, or dizziness.

Heart Valve Disease: See symptoms listed under "Heart Failure."

High Blood Pressure: Mention any problems with shortness of breath, chest pain or other symptoms of heart failure (see "Heart Failure" entry in this list), change in vision, new problems with weakness or numbness, dizziness, lightheadedness, ringing in the ears, nose bleed, rapid heart beat, confusion, and nausea or vomiting.

HIV (Human Immunodeficiency Virus): Indicate any symptoms similar to those of the flu, such as fatigue, fever, headaches, aching muscles, sore throat, or swollen glands. Also note any white patches on the tongue, shortness of breath, diarrhea, nausea or vomiting, night sweats, cough, pain and numbness in the feet, change in thinking ability, or purple spots on the skin.

Hypothyroidism (underactive thyroid gland): Describe any difficulty tolerating cold temperatures, dryness of skin, hair loss, constipation, lack of energy, hoarseness, puffiness around the eyes, or decreased hearing. Symptoms of excess thyroid medication and *hyperthyroidism* (overactive thyroid gland) include feeling intolerant of heat, anxiety, palpitations, and losing weight with diarrhea.

Inflammatory Bowel Disease (ulcerative colitis and Crohn's disease): These are diseases associated with inflammation of the intestines. Note any abdominal pain, diarrhea containing blood or mucus, fever, loss of appetite, weight loss, joint pains, or rash.

Irregular Heart Beat (such as atrial fibrillation): Describe any palpitations, dizziness, chest pain, shortness of breath. Mention any symptoms associated with stroke and heart failure (see "Brain Disorders" and "Heart Failure" entries in this list).

Liver Disease, including Hepatitis (inflammation of the liver) and Cirrhosis (scarring of the liver): Tell the doctor about any change in appetite, fever, nausea or vomiting, joint pains, muscle aches, dark urine, abdominal pain, yellowing of the skin, weight loss, fatigue, itchy skin, tendency to bruise, or fluid buildup in the abdomen .

Lyme Disease: An infection transmitted by ticks. Tell the doctor about any rashes, headaches, fatigue, flu-like symptoms, listlessness, drooping of one side of the face, joint pains, swelling, confusion, numbness, or weakness in limbs.

Lung Cancer: Describe cough, coughing up blood, shortness of breath, or hoarseness. If the cancer has spread to other parts of the body, describe other symptoms, such as bone pain, new weakness, or any symptoms listed under the entry in this list entitled "Brain Disorders."

Myasthenia Gravis: An autoimmune disorder causing muscle weakness. Note any double vision, eyelid drooping, weakness of muscles of face and limbs, problems chewing, difficulty speaking or swallowing, or lack of energy.

Obesity: Skin infections, joint pains, symptoms of diabetes mellitus (see entry in this list), varicose veins, gallstones, shortness of breath, difficulty sleeping, symptoms of high blood pressure (see entry in this list), symptoms of coronary artery disease (see entry in this list).

Parkinson's Disease: This is a degenerative disease of specific neurons in the brain that are important for smooth, controlled movements of parts of the body. Note symptoms of shaking of limbs, stiffness of movements of arms and legs, slowness or lack of movement of limbs, difficulty beginning a movement, stooped or unsteady walking with shuffling steps, falling frequently, monotonous sounding speech, confusion, dry eyes, drooling, difficulty swallowing, constipation, and difficulty sleeping.

Peptic ulcer: Describe any symptoms of nausea, vomiting, vomiting up blood, or abdominal pain.

Prostate Enlargement or Cancer: Describe urinary symptoms, such as feelings of urgency, dribbling, thinner or decreased urinary flow, or blood in urine. In the case of prostate cancer, mention any new problems with back pain, pains in limbs, limb weakness or numbness, or loss of bowel control.

Sciatica: This is a general term used to describe a radiating pain down the leg associated with spinal problems, such as a slipped disc pressing on a nerve.

Seizures (Epilepsy): See "Loss of Consciousness, Fainting, or Seizures" in Chapter 3 for information on seizures.

Systemic Lupus Erythematosus: A disease in which the body's defense system attacks different parts of the body. Tell the doctor about any joint pains, fever, rash, change in mood, vision difficulties, swelling in the limbs, hair loss, susceptibility to bruising, sores in the mouth or nose, chest pain, shortness of breath, palpitations, muscle pains or weakness, change in appetite, nausea, vomiting, abdominal pain, confusion, or seizures.

Urinary Tract Infection: Describe any pain or burning that occurs when you urinate, how often urination occurs, urgency to urinate, amount of urine produced, and fever.

What Was that Medication Called?

Doctors see this problem over and over again. A tremendous amount of time is wasted when doctors and patients try to recall and clarify the names and doses of the medications being taken. You may be heading for the danger zone if you think you can completely depend on your doctor to figure this out. For one thing, medications are often changed between office visits. Perhaps your doctor directed changes over the phone in response to hearing about a side effect or when she heard your symptoms were not getting any better. This may not be documented in the record and it certainly will not be listed in the prior office notes. Maybe another doctor changed the dose or introduced another medication. Try to remember if you made any medication changes without notifying the doctor or whether you ran out of medication and did not take your regular dose.

Before each office visit, review your medications and list them under the medication section of Form 11. Specify the name of the drug, the total dose per day, and exactly how many milligrams (mg.) you take during each part of the day. Bring the actual pills and labeled pill containers to the office, so that your doctor can confirm that you are taking the proper dosage. Consider keeping a list of your medications in your wallet or purse, including the dosages and times they are taken. This information will then be available automatically at the time of your office visits or during emergencies.

As discussed in Chapter 7, many medications have potentially dangerous drug interactions, and keeping a list of the medications you are taking allows your doctor to review the combinations being taken.

Medication Side Effects

The medication section of Form 11 also places emphasis on drug side effects and how well you feel while taking a drug. Sometimes, new symptoms occur coincidentally during the time a medication is introduced. Clues that the medication is responsible include noting that the symptoms occurs at a specific time after taking the medication, worsening of the symptom when dosage is increased, and reduction of the symptom when the medication is reduced or discontinued. However, if you are taking more than one medication, it can be difficult to identify which drug is responsible for any side effect. In fact, irrespective of the specific medication introduced, the more drugs you are taking, the higher the chances that you will have side effects from the next drug that is introduced. This is why it makes sense for your doctor to reduce the total number of medications you are taking or consider a different combination before abandoning the new drug because of side effects. It may be that the new drug would have been very effective and well-tolerated if used alone or in combination with fewer or different drugs.

Not all side effects of drugs are negative ones. Beyond the desired goal of the treatment, medications can sometimes cause coincidental positive effects as well. Some medications may improve mood or energy levels, an extra benefit that may not have been unexpected. Your doctor may consider these positive effects when deciding which medication is best for you.

Now where did I put those test results?

By the time of a follow-up visit, it is likely that some form of testing has been ordered, such as blood tests or X-rays. Since many of these tests may not have been performed in the doctor's office, test results may not necessarily have been received in the mail or via fax, or placed in your file promptly. A typical office scenario consists of the patient asking the doctor "Did you receive my blood test results?" The doctor thumbs through the chart and cannot find them in the thick stack of papers comprising the medical record. To help avoid this problem, Form 11 asks you to specify what lab tests were performed since the last encounter, and where and when they were performed. If the Follow-up Visit Form is reviewed by the doctor before you are brought into the office, the doctor has an opportunity to call for a result or look in your office file. This also gives the doctor a chance to think about what needs to be done in light of your test results and what needs to be explained to you.

What Is Most Important to You?

The issues for discussion that are the most important for you are not necessarily the same as the issues that the doctor thinks are the priority. We constantly hear stories about doctors who do not take the time to truly listen to their patients, investing much more time assessing a blood count rather than how an illness affects a person's life or a person's fears about their medical condition.

Why should discussion of the patient's priorities *not* become as standard as review of a platelet count?

At the author's epilepsy center, we try to bring this issue to the forefront by automatically asking people at each visit "What do you consider to be the main issues for discussion during today's visit?" Placing emphasis on the concerns of people in this way has proved to be highly successful and very gratifying for our patients and our staff.

FORM II

Follow-up Visit

Date of last encounter with the doctor in the office or hospital: _____

If applicable, note what was discussed during any recent telephone conversation with the doctor: _____

_____

_____

_____

Name of Problem: _____

Date of Episode: _____

Description: _____

_____

_____

Medications:

Name of Medication	Total dose (mg.) per day	How medication is administered (# mg. in A.M., # mg. in P.M.)

What changes were made in medication doses since the last visit? _____

_____

_____

Do you believe you are experiencing any side effects from your medications and/or treatments? If so, please specify: _____

_____

_____

_____

_____

Do you believe you are experiencing any positive effects from your treatments? _____

_____

_____

_____

What lab work or X-rays did you have on or since your last visit that need to be discussed during today's visit? When and where were they performed?

_____

_____

_____

_____

What do you believe are the main issues that need to be discussed during today's visit? _____

_____

_____

_____

PART II
Special Situations

CHAPTER 15

Your Child's Medical History

To address the special medical needs and concerns of children, we recommend supplementing the preceding forms with Form 12. This form adds important information that is not emphasized on the adult forms, such as the medical history around the time of the child's birth, growth, and physical and social development. Form 12 also promotes maintaining an ongoing record of commonly administered screening tests, such as testing for lead, and injury prevention methods that your family is using. It concludes with inquiries about psychosocial history. The completed form may be used to anticipate questions that are likely to be asked by the doctor. Alternatively, it can be submitted to the doctor for review before the office visit.

Explanation of Form 12

Form 12 begins with identifying information. This section includes an inquiry as to the child's ethnic background, because some illnesses occur more commonly among specific ethnic or racial groups.

The questions relating to the Chief Complaint and the History of Present Illness are similar to those you would answer for an adult. These questions are most relevant when there is a specific concern that warrants the doctor's attention. The Past Medical History section differs from the questions in the adult form in that it delves into the history before and shortly after birth of the child. This information is not only useful in providing a long-term record of information, but it may alert the doctor to the child's risk of developing future difficulties in both medical and psychological health.

In the section about allergies, list the symptoms observed, the suspected cause, how long the reaction lasted, and how it was treated. Since good nutrition is critical for proper development, the form also emphasizes questions about diet. Indeed, much of Form 12 is devoted to the child's development. Completing these sections will help the doctor determine whether the child's pattern of physical, emotional, and social development fits or deviates from a normal course.

Do not be discouraged if you cannot recall the specific types and dates of immunizations. Consider asking the child's doctor to provide copies of the immunization record and then continue this record on your own as further immunizations are given.

The final portion of Form 12 gives you an opportunity to describe the child's home environment and those who take care of the child. It is also helpful to describe your child's typical day. Remember to complete the Family History and Review of Systems Forms for your child, which are listed in Chapters 5 and 10 respectively.

FORM 12

Child Medical History[9]

Identifying Information

Name: _____

Date of birth: _____

Place of birth: _____

Name of each parent: _____

Child's ethnic background: _____

Are parents living together or separated? _____

If the latter, address and contact information for each: _____

_____

_____

If there is an alternative guardian, please specify: _____

_____

Chief Complaint

In a few words, describe the main problem that led to the current evaluation: _____

_____

_____

_____

9. Adapted in part from *Comprehensive History: Child Patient in Bates' Guide to Physical Examination and History Taking* by L.S Bickley and R.A. Hoekelman, Eds. New York: Lippincott, 1999:39-42.

Who is raising the concerns: child, parent, other family member, teacher, other? _____

_____

History of Present Illness: In addition to filling out Form 12, also fill out Form 2, "History of Present Illness" in Chapter 1.

Past Medical History
1. Birth History
Before Delivery

Did the mother have any illnesses, infections, or bleeding during the pregnancy with this child? _____

_____

Did the mother smoke during the pregnancy? If so, how much? _____

_____

Did the mother drink alcohol during the pregnancy? If so, how much? ____

_____

Did the mother use prescription drugs during the pregnancy? If so, specify?

_____

Did the mother use illegal drugs during the pregnancy? If so, specify? _____

_____

How long was the pregnancy? _____

During Delivery

Were there any difficulties during labor? _____

_____

How long was the labor? _____

Was the delivery a normal, spontaneous vaginal delivery? If the delivery occurred with the use of forceps or by cesarean, why were they needed? ____

_____

_____

What kinds of medications or techniques, such as epidural anesthesia, were used to relieve pain? _____

_____

Were there any complications during the delivery? _____

_____

Is the child a twin? If so, what was the order of births? _____

_____

After delivery

What did the baby weigh at birth? _____

Was there a need to resuscitate the baby because of failure to breathe adequately? _____

What was the *Apgar* score? (Rating scale up to score of 10 based on the infant's appearance, assessed immediately after birth). _____

Were there any difficulties in the areas of feeding, breathing, blue lips, jaundice (abnormal yellow skin color), anemia, seizures, abnormal physical appearance, or infections? If so, specify. _____

_____

_____

Did the child come home from the hospital with the mother? _____

Were there any difficulties in feeding or sleeping? _____

Were there any problems with excessive crying or colic? _____

2. Childhood Illnesses

In addition to illness to be listed in the Past Medical History section on Form 3 in Chapter 4, list whether the child has been evaluated by a doctor for other symptoms, including dizziness, headaches, slow development, seizures, sleeping problems, nausea or vomiting, feeding problems, learning difficulties, genetic diseases, birth defects, skin problems, psychiatric illness, fainting, muscle weakness, infections, accidents and injuries, gastrointestinal problems, or problems with eyes, ears, throat, skin or other parts of the body. If so, specify.

_____

_____

_____

_____

_____

_____

Hospitalizations

List any operations and hospitalizations or emergency room visits for accidents and injuries. _____

_____

_____

Allergies

List any allergic illnesses or symptoms, including eczema, rashes, runny nose, asthma, food allergies, and allergic reactions to insect bites. _____

_____

_____

_____

3. Feeding History
Infancy

What method of feeding was used when the child was a baby? Was the child breastfed? If so, until when? Was the child fed with a bottle, or a combination of breastfeeding and bottle feeding? _____

_____

If formula was used, what type? _____

When were solid foods introduced? _____

Were vitamin or iron supplements given? _____

Was there any nausea, vomiting, diarrhea, or abdominal pain? _____

Were there any problems with weight or growth? _____

_____

Childhood

What does the child eat? What foods are preferred and what foods are disliked? _____

_____

_____

_____

How much does the child eat per day? _____

_____

_____

4. Growth and Development

Are there any problems with physical growth? _____

Are there any concerns about slow or inadequate development of thinking
function or walking? _____

_____

Are there any concerns about behavior? _____

_____

_____

Are there any problems with weight? _____

For children 2 to 4 years old

How does the child socialize—for example, does the child make eye
contact? Does the child approach other children? Is the child aggressive?
Does the child share? _____

_____

_____

Does the child respond to her name being called? How does the child
communicate? Does she point or speak in words or sounds that are similar
to words? Does the child look for a response to what she says? How does
the child ask for something she wants? Is the child easily frustrated if not
understood? _____

_____

_____

Are the child's behaviors rigid—for example, does the child need to hold a
toy at all times, seem mesmerized, or want to watch only one video over and
over? _____

_____

Does the child avoid being touched? Is the child very disturbed by noises?

_____

_____

Does the child play with the same toys all the time? Does the child play with the toys appropriately? _____

_____

_____

For children up to 4 years old who are speaking

Can the child give an answer to a "Who, What, When, Where, or Why" question? _____

_____

Physical Growth

What were the approximate weight and height at the following times:

Age (years)	Weight	Height
1	_____	_____
2	_____	_____
5	_____	_____
10	_____	_____

Was there any slow or rapid gain in height or weight? _____

When did the baby teeth begin to appear? _____

When did the baby teeth begin to be lost? _____

When did the permanent teeth begin to come in? _____

Developmental Milestones

At what ages did the child achieve the following milestones in development?

Milestone	Age (months or years)
Held up head while lying on the stomach	_____
Rolled over from front to back and back to front	_____
Sat with support	_____
Sat alone	_____
Stood with support	_____
Stood alone	_____

Walked with support _____

Walked alone _____

Said first word _____

Said first combination of words _____

Said first sentences _____

Tied own shoes _____

Dressed without help _____

Was toilet trained _____

Walked up steps _____

Walked down steps _____

Pedaled a tricycle _____

Others you would like to mention:

_____

_____

_____

Social Development
Sleep

How many hours of sleep does the child get per day? _____

Are there any problems with nightmares or terrors when the child is not asleep? _____

_____

Does the child sleepwalk? _____

Toilet Training

When was toilet training achieved? _____

Are there any problems with loss of urine or bowel movement during sleep?

_____

Are there any problems with loss or urine or bowel movements during waking hours? _____

_____

Speech

How well does the child communicate? _____

Approximately how many words are in the child's the current vocabulary?

_____

Are there any speech abnormalities, such as hesitation, stuttering, or lisp? ___

_____

Personality

How does the child relate to other members of the family? _____

_____

How does the child relate to peers? _____

_____

What activities does the child engage in alone? _____

_____

What activities does the child engage in with other children? _____

_____

What interests does the child have? _____

_____

Describe the child's personality. _____

_____

What are the child's major positive attributes and skills? _____

_____

_____

How is the child's self-esteem? _____

_____

Discipline

How is the child disciplined? _____

How well does this work? _____

Are there any problems with temper tantrums? _____

Are there any problems with aggressive behavior? _____

_____

Schooling

Describe the child's experience, if applicable, in:

Day care _____

_____

Nursery school _____

_____

Kindergarten _____

_____

Early elementary school _____

_____

How is the child doing in school? _____

_____

Have any concerns been raised by the school staff? ____

_____

Sexuality

What has the child been taught about sexuality, masturbation, sexual body parts, and sexually transmitted diseases? _____

_____

_____

5. Health Maintenance
Immunizations

Type of Vaccine	Date or Age it was Last Received	Negative Reactions
Tetanus		
Pertussis		
Diphtheria		
Polio		
Measles		
Rubella		
Mumps		

Influenza _____ _____

Hepatitis B _____ _____

Haemophilus Influenzae _____ _____

Pneumococcus _____ _____

Lyme _____ _____

Chicken Pox (Varicella) _____ _____

Other: _____ _____

Other: _____ _____

6. Screening Procedures

This information can be obtained from the child's doctor. A problem may be listed more than once.

Screening Test	Age or Date	Result
Blood Pressure	_____	_____
Vision Testing	_____	_____
Hearing Testing	_____	_____
Tuberculin Testing	_____	_____
Blood Lead Levels	_____	_____
Urinalysis	_____	_____
Blood Counts	_____	_____
Tests for any metabolic or genetic disorders, such as PKU	_____	_____
Other	_____	_____
	_____	_____

7. Safety and Injury Prevention

Are safety-approved car seats and seat belts always used? _____

Is a helmet worn whenever riding a bicycle? _____

Are there any guns in the house? _____

If so, how are they stored away from the child? _____

Are there smoke and carbon monoxide detectors in the house? _____

What safety precautions are in place to prevent:
Burn injuries from a stove or heater _____

Drowning in a pool _____

Choking on small items _____

Scalding from a stove or heater? _____

8. Psychosocial History

Who lives in the home and what are their relationships with the child? ____

_____

_____

Describe the child's typical day. _____

_____

_____

What other extended family members is the child regularly exposed to? ___

_____

How is the health of others living or working in the home? _____

_____

What are the work schedules of the parents? _____

_____

_____

Who attends to the child after school? _____

What support is available from relatives, friends, and people in the neighborhood? What is the religious and cultural background of the family? Are there any specific beliefs about health care and treatment that the doctor should be aware of? _____

_____

_____

_____

CHAPTER 16

The Psychiatric Consultation

"Through most of my adult life, when I was either manic – doing so many bizarre, off-the-wall things – or depressed, taking to my bed for weeks refusing to see anyone, I kept thinking, 'There must be something, something I could take that would make this all go away, that would make me stop behaving this way.' … I knew from a very young age that there was something very wrong with me, but I thought it was just that I was not a good person, that I did not try hard enough. As with many people, the overt symptoms of my manic-depressive illness did not show themselves until my late teens. And that was with a manic episode. From that time on, until I was diagnosed at the age of 35, I rode a wild roller coaster from agitated, out-of-control highs to disabling, often suicidal lows."

PATTY DUKE
A Brilliant Madness: Living with Manic-Depressive Illness

The Adult Consultation

When my doctor recommended a psychiatrist, I got really angry. He said it would be helpful because I was feeling sad and tearful, but he must think I'm crazy.

When a doctor recommends seeing a psychiatrist, many people feel upset, embarrassed, or angry. People may feel the doctor is minimizing their medical problem and physical pain, or is essentially telling them that *it is all in their heads*. Unfortunately, there is still a great deal of stigma and misunderstanding associated with psychiatric consultation. Typically, a primary care doctor refers a person to a psychiatrist because of important concerns about depression, anxiety, mood swings, or other conditions. Psychiatrists are medical doctors who specialize in the evaluation and treatment of such conditions. Since there now are many effective treatments for psychiatric conditions, it is all the more critical that a careful evaluation be performed.

Primary care doctors who recommend psychiatric evaluations may be more attuned to the psychological needs of their patients, and they show their sensitivity to these emotional needs by recommending such a referral. Some primary care doctors prefer to prescribe drugs for psychiatric diagnoses, such as antidepressants, without the involvement of a psychiatrist. We believe this is less than optimal, because proper psychiatric treatment is highly dependent on having expertise in this area. Ideally, a person should have a full psychiatric assessment when psychiatric diagnoses and treatments are initially considered. Once someone is stabilized on a regular medication regimen, he may discuss whether it is advisable to have the primary care doctor take over. Unfortunately, limitations in the availability of psychiatrists and other realities of our current health care system may adversely affect the quality of psychiatric treatment in many areas of the country.

Unlike many medical disorders that can be confirmed by identifying an abnormality on a laboratory test, there is no blood test that can specifically identify or confirm a psychiatric diagnosis. Therefore, the psychiatric interview and examination, which are highly dependant on the interview and examination skills of the psychiatric health care provider, are especially crucial. Currently in most of the United States, only psychiatrists, nurse practitioners, and other medical doctors are able to prescribe medication. Only a psychiatrist is trained to assess the medical aspects of a psychiatric history and examination, although social workers, psychologists, and nurse practitioners can perform a number of the aspects of a psychiatric interview.

An initial consultation with a psychiatrist is typically similar to the first meeting with other types of doctors. A typical interview includes questions about the presenting problems, the history and symptoms of the present illness, as well as past medical history and family history. In addition, you will be asked about any past psychiatric history and your personal history, including childhood and development, relationships with family and friends, educational and occupational history, the use of substances, including tobacco, drugs, and alcohol, and life events associated with emotional trauma and losses. Because a number of psychiatric problems appear to have family associations, being able to provide well-organized background information about your family history is very important. Form 13A will help you determine if there have been any psychiatric issues in your family. It would be advisable for you to fill out this form and bring it with you to your first appointment with a psychiatrist.

The typical initial psychiatric interview lasts approximately 45 to 90 minutes, although several follow-up interviews may be needed to complete the evaluation. Psychiatric examiners vary in their amount of note-taking during the psychiatric interview, although most do take some notes. A skillful psychiatrist puts a person at ease during a consultation, so that most of the meeting is experienced as an informal discussion of a person's problems, experiences, and life history. The most formal part of a psychiatric examination is called the *Mental Status Exam*. This is an examination by a psychiatrist of an individual's cognitive (thinking) functions. Sometimes, people question or become troubled about why the psychiatrist asks silly-sounding questions such as "Do you ever hear voices?" or "What is today's date?" or "Name three presidents." These questions are not designed to be insulting; they are necessary because they may bring out difficulties some people are having in their ability to think clearly.

During a mental status examination, the psychiatrist systematically examines different aspects of the person's presentation. These include an assessment of:

- The individual's general appearance — for example, coming to the appointment completely unkempt
- Behaviors associated with movements — for example, agitation, slowness, or shaking of limbs
- The nature of speech — for example, the hesitancy and low volume that may be seen in depression, or the pressured speech that may be observed in a state called *mania*
- Abnormalities in thought content, such as delusions (fixed, false beliefs despite evidence to the contrary) or in the process of how ideas are expressed, such as illogically jumping from one thought to another.

Typical Mental Status Questions

During the psychiatric mental status examination, the doctor may routinely ask questions about:

- Your mood and emotional state
- Thoughts that you may be preoccupied with
- Suspicious thoughts about others
- Any strange or unusual ideas that seem unrelated to reality
- Thoughts about harming yourself or others
- Obsessions: Unwanted thoughts that are disturbing and repetitively intrude on your thinking
- Hallucinations: Perceiving something that is not really there, such as hearing voices, feeling the sensation of insects crawling on your skin, or seeing images that are not real
- Illusions: Misinterpretations of a true sensory stimulus in the environment — for example, seeing a shadow and thinking it is a bear, or hearing a loud crash and thinking it is a gunshot
- Orientation: You may be asked who you are, where you are, and the date.
- Concentration: You may be asked to recite numbers backwards and forwards.

- Memory: Your short-term memory may be tested by being asked to remember a few items immediately and then to recall those same items after five minutes. Long-term memory may be checked by asking about events that occurred more than several years ago.

- Calculations: You may be asked to perform simple arithmetic.

- Fund of knowledge: You may be asked about current events or simple geography questions.

- Abstract reasoning: Abstraction is the reasoning capacity we should have by our teenage years in order to shift from the specific to the more general. This is often tested by asking someone to interpret proverbs, such as "What does it mean when someone says 'a rolling stone gathers no moss,'" or to describe the similarities between two items.

- Insight: Your ability to recognize that a problem exists and how much you understand the problem.

- Judgment: You may be asked a hypothetical situation, such as "What would you do if you were in a crowded theater and someone suddenly cried fire?"

The Child or Adolescent Consultation

When a recommendation is made for a psychiatric referral for a child or adolescent, parents may feel guilty, worried, or overwhelmed. Alternatively, parents may feel intense anger and humiliation that the referring source feels that a psychiatric evaluation is indicated. These reactions are understandable and should be discussed candidly with a psychiatrist who specializes in children and adolescents. Nonetheless, it is important to acknowledge and examine the kinds of behavioral difficulties that a child is having, in order to ensure that the child receives proper diagnosis and treatment. A child and adolescent psychiatrist is a psychiatrist who has had at least two years of specialized training in child and adolescent psychiatry, and is therefore best equipped to provide the most optimal psychiatric evaluation and treatment of children.

The concerns that often lead a parent to bring a child for a consultation often involve questions such as: "Is my child's emotional and psychological development progressing normally?" Child and adolescent psychiatrists are quite knowledgeable about normal development and can often provide significant reassurance for parents. Other concerns that are appropriately handled by child and adolescent psychiatrists concern how a child interacts with peers, issues of underachievement in school, or evaluation of depressed mood. Psychiatric evaluation should also be considered in the presence of any symptoms listed below, particularly if they last more than two weeks. Form 13B lists situations where it is advisable to consider a psychiatric consultation for a child or adolescent. Use this form to make notes to remind yourself what to tell the child's doctor.

Unlike the psychiatric evaluation of an adult, the evaluation of a child is more involved and lasts several hours. The psychiatrist obtains a detailed history of the current problem as well as the child's past psychiatric and developmental history. It is helpful if the parent brings records of prior psychological or psychiatric evaluations, as well as the child's report cards or other educational reports. The family psychiatric history mentioned above is also important here. A child should also be prepared, in a matter-of-fact way, and told that they will be meeting with a doctor who will be talking with them about whatever problems or concerns they may be having. Sometimes it is helpful to explain to anxious, younger children that the doctor is a special kind of doctor who talks to children about how they feel—not the kind of doctor who gives shots.

After obtaining a detailed history from the parent, the child psychiatrist interviews the child, usually without the parent present. The psychiatrist will try to engage the child and help him feel comfortable in the interview situation. Toys, drawings, and games can be useful tools in evaluating the child. Alternatively, the psychiatrist may simply talk with the child. As with adults, the psychiatrist will ask questions in order to assess a variety of areas of functioning, including but not limited to:

- The child's overall mood and any symptoms of anxiety
- Inattention, hyperactivity, and other aspects of behavior
- The child's thought patterns and content of thought, including the possible presence of any unusual preoccupations or obsessions, or problems with reality testing, such as auditory or visual hallucinations
- The child's thinking abilities and language skills
- Specific questions for adolescents if there are issues about substance abuse or if the adolescent is sexually active. Likewise, concerns about traumatic events, such as possible sexual or physical abuse bring up different sets of questions.

When the interview with the child is completed, the psychiatrist meets again with the parents and discusses his findings and recommendations. Depending on the age of the child or adolescent, the psychiatrist may invite the child or adolescent to sit in on the discussion with the parents. Some of the common conditions or diagnoses that the psychiatrist may discuss include:

- **Attention Deficit Hyperactivity Disorder (ADHD):** A disorder characterized by problems in attention, impulsivity, and distractibility. Hyperactivity may or may not be present.

- **Oppositional Defiant Disorder (ODD):** A disorder associated with persistent hostile, defiant, or uncooperative behaviors, particularly toward those in authority. These behaviors seriously interfere with a child's functioning within the family and in school.

- **Conduct Disorder:** A disorder with behaviors that violate the rights of others—for example, fighting, bullying, stealing, lying, and fire-setting.

- **Bipolar Disorder:** A disorder with severe mood swings (ranging from highs known as *mania* to lows of *depression*). This disorder is also sometimes referred to as *manic-depressive illness*.

- **Major Depressive Disorder:** A state of serious, persistent sadness that lasts for at least two weeks and is associated with feelings of hopelessness, loss of interest in usual activities, and sometimes thoughts of death, suicide, or suicidal gestures.

- **Anxiety Disorder:** This disorder is marked by excessive worrying that interferes with the child's normal functioning. Examples of subtypes include *Social Phobia* in which there is intense and persistent fear of being in social or performance situations. *Separation Anxiety* is characterized by abnormally intense fear of being separated from parents. *Generalized Anxiety Disorder* is associated with constant worrying over things that do not necessarily warrant such anxiety. *Post-Traumatic Stress Disorder* occurs after exposure to trauma and consists of constantly thinking about the event, experiencing severe anxiety, and avoiding things that remind the child of the event.

- **Obsessive Compulsive Disorder:** *Obsessions* are intrusive thoughts, often of an upsetting nature, such as anxiety about germs or violent images. *Compulsions* are uncontrollable repetitive behaviors resulting from urges to perform a task, such as repetitively washing one's hands, cleaning, or checking things over and over again. This disorder is characterized by both obsessions and compulsions.

- **Eating Disorders:** Examples of eating disorders are *Anorexia Nervosa* (associated with self-starvation and extreme weight loss); *Binge Eating*

Disorder (compulsive overeating); and *Bulimia Nervosa* (associated with cycles of binges and then purges through vomiting or the use of laxatives).

- **Pervasive Developmental Disorders:** These are developmental disabilities associated with problems in communication skills, social interaction, and imaginative activities. There may be associated abnormalities in coordination or thinking abilities. *Autism* is a form of this disorder that includes severe limitations in the range of activities and interests, abnormal patterns of play, unusual responses to lights or sounds, and sometimes repetitive self-injurious body movements. *Asperger's Disorder* is a pervasive developmental disorder associated with high or normal intelligence. Language development is less affected. However, a serious impairment in social interaction is present as well as repetitive behaviors and restrictive interests.

- **Schizophrenia:** This is a severe psychiatric disorder that is uncommon in childhood. Children with schizophrenia may appear different from adults with this illness, which may begin by having trouble confusing reality and fantasy. The child may see things and hear voices that are not real (hallucinations), experience paranoia, psychosis, and delusions (see definitions in previous adult section) and exhibit disorganized language and behavior, among other symptoms.

- **Enuresis (bedwetting):** Bedwetting is not a disease, but rather a common symptom in childhood. The child may urinate in inappropriate places during the day or wet the bed at night, although she has already attained control during toilet training. Enuresis occurs past the typical age of toilet training.

- **Encopresis (soiling):** Encopresis is the repeated passage of feces by a child over the age of four into inappropriate places, such as the underwear, either purposely or unintentionally.

Understanding the nature and reasoning behind the psychiatric evaluation should be helpful to you, if you or a family member undergoes such an assessment. If you have concerns about any part of the psychiatric evaluation, it is important for you to openly voice your concerns.

Your Family's Psychiatric History

To your knowledge, has any member of your family—including your parents, siblings, aunts, uncles, or grandparents—had any of the problems listed below? Specify your relationship to each person and whether the individual was on your mother or father's side of the family.

	Relationship to Self	Mother's Side	Father's Side
Nervous Breakdown			
Depression			
Severe Mood Swings			
Suicide			
Suicide Attempt			
Bipolar (Manic Depressive)			
Psychiatric Hospitalization			
Schizophrenia			
Alcoholism			
Drug Abuse			
Committed a Serious Crime			
Attention Deficit Hyperactivity Disorder			
Learning Disabilities			
Autism			
Mental Retardation			
Other			

When to Think About Getting a Consultation with a Child and Adolescent Psychiatrist

Let your doctor know if your child has any of these symptoms:

Behaves like the opposite sex _____

Can't sit still or acts as if driven by a motor _____

Has difficulty paying attention or is easily distracted _____

Starts physical fights or is aggressive _____

Is frequently oppositional and/or defiant _____

Is excessively tearful or anxious _____

Has many physical complaints without medical causes (e.g. stomachaches, headaches, or problems with eyes) _____

Has unusual ideas or odd behaviors _____

Is often irritable or depressed _____

Talks about suicide or topics associated with death _____

Has difficulty learning and/or organizing schoolwork or homework_____

Has difficulty making friends or relating with other people _____

Drinks alcohol, uses marijuana and/or uses other illegal drugs _____

Worries excessively about getting fat or thinks he/she is overweight but really isn't _____

Has experienced a emotionally traumatic event (e.g. divorce, death or serious illness) _____

Has heard sounds or voices that aren't there _____

Can't get his/her mind off particular thoughts _____

Is extremely active, abnormally cheerful and needs only a few hours of sleep

_____

Has had a significant decline in academic performance or decrease in socialization _____

Appears excessively fatigued or trouble sleeping _____

Refuses or avoids school _____

Displays marked mood swings _____

Lies and steals _____

CHAPTER 17

Preparing the Medical Evaluation for People with Impaired Thinking

"My wish is to see handicapped people helped by love, positive thinking, increased programs, and a caring public. Society must open doors
to the handicapped and be concerned with their problems. The handicapped must play an active role in our society. People who are different should not be shunned.... I address my new friends as the person
I am; I no longer find myself making excuses for who I am. No
longer do I tell them about my handicaps, although at times an occasional astute observer makes note of a facial asymmetry.

I do not become dismayed and wallow in self-pity. Instead, I forge
ahead with the hope that I will help others as I have been helped. I
want to encourage them by saying, 'Believe in your dream; image it,
and persevere. The victory will be yours.'"

BEATRICE C. ENGSTRAND
The Gift of Healing: A Legacy of Hope

Most of the forms in this book are designed to be completed by competent
individuals. However, some conditions affecting the brain, such as mental retardation, developmental disabilities, severe head injuries, and degenerative
neurologic diseases, can cause problems in thinking and language function.
People with these types of conditions need others to complete the forms for
them. A supplementary form that is useful in such cases is Form 14, which establishes a baseline for future reference about intellectual impairments,
speech and language limitations, and difficulties in neurologic function. Form
14 can be completed by close family members or staff members at facilities
where such individuals reside. The authors have used this form at numerous
clinics for people with developmental disabilities and have found staff and
family to be very enthusiastic about providing information.

Explanation of Form 14

The first question in Form 14 asks for information about any known causes
for thinking impairments and reminds the doctor to think about what may
have caused the problem. For example, while some causes of mental retardation relate to lack of oxygen at birth or severe infections in early childhood,
doctors should not forget about the possibility of genetic causes.

Sometimes, brain disturbances are accompanied by problems in behavior, such as screaming, throwing things, grabbing, spitting, being withdrawn, and other negative behaviors. Other medical conditions and treatments can also cause changes in behavior and, therefore, recording behaviors at baseline is crucial for verifying that a change has indeed occurred.

Most of Form 14 is self-explanatory and follows the typical order of information collected during a neurologic examination. The first series of questions relating to language and thinking function helps the doctor understand a person's ability to communicate and gives a clue as to how an individual relates to others. The next questions ask about functions that pertain to the individual nerves that control the senses and parts of the head and neck region. Knowing about weakness, numbness, or coordination difficulties, as noted in subsequent sections, alerts the doctor to specific neurologic problems.

> Mr. Sutton is a 42-year-old man with Down's syndrome (a genetic disorder associated with mental retardation) who moved to a new supervised residential facility. Recently, Mr. Sutton's functioning appears to be deteriorating. For example, when he applies toothpaste to the toothbrush he seems confused about what to do next. He needs vigorous assistance in getting dressed and in bathing. Fortunately, good documentation from prior records reveals that in the past, Mr. Sutton was able to brush his teeth independently, get dressed on his own, and take a shower with minimal assistance. With the evidence of decline in Mr. Sutton's functioning, Dr. Sutherling looks for possible causes. He suspects Alzheimer's disease, a common complication of Down's syndrome. After excluding other possible reasons, Dr. Sutherland prescribes one of several recently introduced medications that are used to slow down the decline associated with Alzheimer's disease.

People with developmental disabilities or intellectual impairments often have difficulty expressing their own medical needs. Signs and symptoms can be easily overlooked. Gradual, but significant changes in function can be missed unless a rigorous method of tracking observations of the individual is used. People who live in supervised residences commonly move from one facility to another, and prior medical records are often difficult to attain or contain scanty documentation. Using an organized method of documenting the functioning of the individual provides a crucial reference point for future health-care providers to track the health and activity levels of such patients.

Checklist for People with Moderate Impairments in Intellectual Functioning

Name: _____ Date: _____

Intellectual Function Impairment

Are there any known causes of intellectual function impairment? _____

_____

_____

Behavior

How does the person behave? Specify if there are difficulties with screaming inappropriately, talking excessively, temper tantrums, or other negative behaviors. _____

_____

_____

Speech and Language, and Thinking Function

Please describe the person's speech and language. What sounds, phrases or sentences can the person vocalize? _____

_____

Can the person name items, repeat things being said, and understand what is being said? _____

Can the person write or read? _____

Does the person's speech make sense? _____

Can the person attend to his or her appearance? _____

Does the person laugh or cry without control? Does the crying or laughter occur suddenly and without reason? _____

Is the person oriented as to person, place and time? Can they remember things? _____

Can the person perform any mathematical calculations? _____

How complex a command can the person follow? _____

_____

What activities of daily living can the person perform with or without assistance? _____

_____

_____

Does the person appear to have hallucinations or delusions? _____

Does the person appear depressed? _____

Does the person tend to repeat sounds or phrases inappropriately when speaking? _____

Cranial Nerves

How is the person's vision? _____

Does the person have double vision? _____

Are there abnormal eye movements? _____

Is there any drooping of one side of the face? _____

How is the person's hearing? _____

Is there problem with swallowing? _____

Can the person shrug his shoulders? Can the person turn his head from side to side? _____

Can the person stick out his or her tongue? _____

Motor

How is the strength in the right arm? _____

How is the strength in the left arm? _____

How is the strength in the right leg? _____

How is the strength in the left leg? _____

Does the person have rigid tone in one or more limbs of the body? _____

_____

Are there any sudden abnormal movements, such as twisting movements, stretching movements, jerking movements, tremors or shaking movements?

_____

_____

Sensory

Does the person have difficulty feeling things in any part of the body?
Please specify where. _____

_____

Coordination and Gait

Can the person walk? How do they walk? _____

_____

_____

Can the person sit upright on a flat surface, such as his or her bed? _____

_____

CHAPTER 18

Whose Life is it Anyway? – Preparing Advance Directives

What would happen if you suddenly became very ill and were unable to express or make decisions about how you wanted to be treated? What if you were not able to indicate whether you wanted life-sustaining measures? For example, if you were connected to a respirator or receiving electric shocks to your chest to treat severely irregular heart rhythms. While some individuals would want everything possible to be done—regardless of how dire or irreversible the illness—others might feel that their quality of life would be so impaired that they would not want extraordinary measures to be used to sustain their life.

Waiting for a catastrophic event to occur before thinking about these decisions may lead to the possibility that your preferences will not be known and if known, they will not necessarily be honored. Alternatively, considering dire possibilities before they happen provides a crucial opportunity to express your wishes about these matters to your family and your physicians. Two important documents known as the *Living Will* and the *Health Care Power of Attorney* can enable you to state your directions in advance. Therefore, they are called *Advance Directives*. Advance directives enable the voice of the person to be heard in the discussion of care, even after the capacity to do so has been lost.

The Living Will

The Living Will is one type of advance directive. This is a document that allows you to express your wishes about using or withholding life-sustaining treatments in the event of a terminal condition from which your primary health care provider has determined you have no reasonable chance of recovery. Living wills have limitations because some of the terms used in them, such as *terminal*, may be up to interpretation in given circumstances. Some living wills include checklists of specific eventualities, although it is difficult to enumerate all possible specific medical circumstances.

The provisions of a living will differ from state to state, and you should consult an attorney to be sure that the document you sign reflects the law in your state. You may also obtain generic samples of living wills from a number of places on the Internet by typing in "living will" into the search feature; a good example is:

http://www.chron.com/content/chronicle/health/forms/livingwill.html

Health Care Power of Attorney

The Health Care Power of Attorney, also known as the *Health Care Proxy*, is the second type of advance directive. In the event that you become incapacitated and are unable to convey your wishes about medical treatment, this document specifically names the person you authorize to make health care-related decisions on your behalf and gives that person the *legal* authority to do so. The *proxy* (the person you select) should be someone close to you who would be the most likely to execute the best decisions on your behalf, given any specific circumstances. It is important to confer with the appointed person in advance and discuss your wishes in detail in order to ensure that she is willing to assume the role of proxy and will make the decisions that you would want. It is also advisable to select an alternate proxy, should the first person become unavailable to serve in this role.

In the event you suffer an illness where the proxy is needed, she will confer with your health care providers and make decisions about the following:

- Diagnosis and treatment options
- Request additional consultations
- Refuse life-sustaining measures (in some states)
- Order that you be transferred to another facility
- Become involved in the informed consent process before tests or treatments are administered

As with the living will, you should check the details of your health care proxy with an attorney to be sure it is consistent with the laws of the state in which you live. You may also obtain generic samples of health care proxy forms at a number of places on the internet by typing in "health care proxy" into the search feature; a good example (but specifically for the state of New York) is:

http://www.health.state.ny.us/nysdoh/hospital/healthcareproxy/form.htm

Preparation is Your Best Insurance

Unfortunately, many people wait for a crisis before they begin considering advance directives, mistakenly believing that these issues are only applicable to the very sick, elderly, or dying. Yet, unforeseen circumstances, such as devastating injury or profound confusion due to medications or other causes, can afflict the youngest and healthiest among us. Therefore, preparing for the possibility of losing your decision-making capability is the best way to ensure that your health care wishes will be honored in the event of a future problem.

Stating your wishes in advance does not deny you the right to make decisions about your health care. The wishes stated in advance directives go into effect only in the event you lose your capacity to make decisions for yourself. Therefore, these documents do *not* mean loss of control over your current medical decision-making. In addition, advance directives can be changed at any time and as frequently as desired. With a health care proxy in place, you and your proxy will be able to request or refuse treatment of any kind.

Which Directive Should Take Priority?

There are significant differences between living wills and health care proxy appointments. Living wills are static documents that attempt to anticipate medical events that have not yet occurred. Health care proxies make decisions for people when they are unable to make decisions for themselves. This means your proxy can respond to medical conditions that are not terminal. Health care proxies are people who know the values and wishes of the ill or disabled person, and they can communicate with health care providers and respond to changing medical conditions.

While a living will is a static piece of paper, the health care proxy is an actual person who is more flexible and able to respond to ever-changing conditions. The proxy can confer with health care providers, the person's family, and colleagues. Living wills try to anticipate eventualities, but when they are applied to a specific medical situation, they may elicit concern that the person never really meant it in the way it might be applied. The proxy can make informed decisions specific to the individual circumstances, whereas depending on a living will means interpretation of the person's wishes by medical professionals based on a document rather than by someone who has been entrusted with decision-making. To avoid potential conflict between the proxy's instructions and stipulations of the living will, the use of both documents is not recommended. If both are used, it should be specified in advance which one should take priority. A living will should be used when no appropriate person is available to be appointed proxy.

Where to Obtain Advance Directive Forms

Most medical centers and nursing facilities have standard advance directive forms available. Although an attorney is not needed to complete advance directive documents, a lawyer's advice on individual state laws on the matter may be helpful. Some states require two witnesses, and some ask for advance directive documents to be notarized.

For further information about advance directives, an excellent guide *Managing Health Care Decisions for Others: A Guide to Being a Health Care Proxy or Surrogate*, is available by contacting the Division of Bioethics, Montefiore Medical Center, Albert Einstein College of Medicine, 111 E. 210th Street, Bronx, NY 10467-2490.

PART III

Questions for the Doctor

CHAPTER 19

Not Asking About Test Results
Is Out of the Question

"The next morning I was in a radiology office in New York. The technicians strapped me to a table and then put a tube in my rear end. As they poured a chalky liquid inside me and pumped gas into me so that my bowel would show up in a photograph, they were also turning me slowly around and around on the table so that the barium liquid would go all the way through my bowels, making it possible to get pictures at a lot of different angles.

During my days at 'Saturday Night Live,' I had been photographed by Scavullo for the cover of *Rolling Stone* and by Richard Avedon for the Gilda Live billboard at the Winter Garden Theatre, but I had never had a photo session quite like this."

GILDA RADNER
It's Always Something

When I heard that they saw a spot on the CAT scan, I was so confused and frightened that I could not ask one single question. Yet, the doctor did not seem to be concerned. When I got home, I was mad at myself for not asking questions about what he thinks it is.

Hearing about a test result from the doctor can be anxiety-provoking and overwhelming even before a diagnosis is generated. Many people get flustered when receiving test results, then kick themselves later for failing to ask important questions. Organizing your questions before you receive test results can prepare you for this discussion with the doctor and raise the chances you will understand what the test results really mean.

Questions to Ask Your Doctor About Test Results

1. What do the test results mean?

2. If the test shows an abnormality, what are the chances that there really is no abnormality but the test shows a false positive result?

3. If the test comes back normal, what are the chances that there really is an abnormality but the test came back falsely negative?

4. Is it worth backing up this test with repeat testing in the future or having a different test?

5. What are the risks and benefits of any other possible tests?

6. What diagnoses does this test result point to, and which suspected diagnoses does it go against?

7. How seriously is the doctor concerned with the test result? What are the implications of the result?

8. What is the worst possibility that this test result could mean?

9. Where can I learn more about this test and the meaning of the results?

10. Does this test result mean I should take any special precautions or change my lifestyle?

Explanation of the Questions

The first question "What does the test result mean?" is a reminder to insist on receiving a clear explanation about the results. Insist on a repeat explanation in simple language if the doctor uses medical words you do not understand.

How Good is the Test?

Questions 2 and 3 concern the quality of the test performed. When we undergo a test, we tend to think of the results as positive or negative, abnormal or normal, and we want to believe that the test is definitive. In fact, tests used in medicine vary greatly in their accuracy, and the determination as to whether a result is normal or abnormal may not always be clear-cut. The quality of the test is often described in terms of its sensitivity and its specificity. *Sensitivity* refers to the ability of the test to identify as abnormal a result that is truly abnormal. In fact, no test is 100 percent sensitive, which means that some individuals with an abnormality have test results that are called *normal*. *Specificity* refers to how well a test avoids mislabeling a normal result as abnormal. When undergoing a test, it is reasonable to inquire about the quality of the test. If the test comes back positive—leading to the recommendation for more involved testing with perhaps more associated risk or a serious intervention—it is important to learn how likely it is that the test was right or wrong. Alternatively, if the test result is negative, ask your doctor for assurance that the test result is accurate.

To address both positive and negative results, question 4 asks whether further testing is indicated. The risks and benefits of such testing should be discussed. Sometimes, the procedure needed to clarify an earlier test result can be too risky to make it worth pursuing.

How Does the Test Help Determine the Diagnosis?

Ultimately, it is not the test result that affects our lives, but the diagnoses it suggests. Therefore, ask your doctor how the test result will affect his ideas about the diagnosis and how it will alter the selection of other tests.

Do not Assume the Worst!

You may feel extremely anxious when you hear a test result, but you may not be inclined to show your anxiety. You may have certain ideas about dire possibilities that may not have much basis. Bring these ideas out into the open with your doctor. In some cases, you may find out that you were worried for nothing.

Educate Yourself

Many people want to further their understanding of the test results and supplement information given by the doctor. The doctor can often provide useful information about other resources available to learn more about the test results. These may include pamphlets dispensed at the doctor's office, the names and contact information of social service agencies that specialize in disorders related to the test result, or even Internet sites.

Medical Pitfalls (See Appendix B)

Appendix B is adapted from one of the best health care books the authors have encountered. It lists common medical errors related to testing that you should be on the alert for. This is a book well worth reading and it may generate additional questions you will want to ask your doctor.

CHAPTER 20

Questions About Your Diagnosis and When to Get a Second Opinion

> "I opened my very tired and swollen eyes and saw my gynecologist surrounded by several other doctors who were unknown to me standing at the foot of my bed. They asked me quite a few questions about things like the frequency of my urination during the last few weeks, and any unusual thirst and dryness of mouth I might have noticed. Had I felt more than a little fatigued? My answers, all of which were yes, did not seem to surprise these men, who checked their charts and regarded me, as well as each other, with grim, knowing looks. 'Mary,' my doctor said in a falsely reassuring tone, 'you have diabetes.'"
>
> MARY TYLER MOORE
> *After All*

Finally, we arrive at what we have been waiting for: the final verdict, the diagnosis. Diagnoses fall into many different kinds of categories. Sometimes, the given diagnosis is a distinct disease, such as diabetes mellitus or ulcerative colitis. In fact, doctors are taught to explain symptoms based on the fewest number of diagnoses. Sometimes this is feasible, but sometimes symptoms simply cannot be unified under one diagnosis. On some occasions, the diagnosis cannot be condensed beyond a general category of diseases, either because there is insufficient current information to divide the category further, or because the features of the illness are not characteristic of any one disease.

Some diagnoses are classified as a *syndrome*, a collection of symptoms, exams, or test results that tend to go together and require a typical kind of treatment. Some diagnoses have a mostly descriptive quality. For example, *hyponatremia* is a diagnosis that describes a low sodium value. The name does not imply any specific cause.

The toughest part about getting a diagnosis may be the apprehension or anxiety you experience when you meet with the doctor to discuss it. How your doctor explains the diagnosis will have a major effect on your reaction to the information that is delivered. We cannot control how your doctor will reveal a diagnosis to you, but we can suggest that you ensure the doctor explains:

- Name of the diagnosis
- An overview of the speculated causes

- Additional testing required
- Treatment options
- Implications for you and your family
- What to expect over the course of the illness (*prognosis*)
- Suggestions for dealing with the illness

When doctors present information about a diagnosis they should avoid medical terms that are difficult to understand. Although many people feel too inhibited to ask the doctor to clarify words or concepts, understanding the information the doctor gives you about your diagnosis should be your highest priority. One strategy is to summarize out loud in your own words what the doctor has said and see if the doctor agrees with this interpretation. Asking your doctor to draw a picture or diagram may also be helpful.

Remember that no matter how serious the diagnosis, there is always something that can be done, even if finding a cure is not realistic. This includes getting more information, learning about support groups, entering experimental clinical trials, getting another opinion, receiving counseling and rehabilitation, and finding physical or emotional comfort. Sensitive doctors can always find some hopeful or optimistic aspect when presenting even very serious diagnoses. Dismissing a person from the office with the statement "There is nothing further I can do for you" is simply unacceptable.

Even the most devoted and best-intentioned doctors may forget to cover some of these crucial aspects of the diagnosis. Similarly, you may become overwhelmed with confusion and shocked by the diagnosis, and may forget to ask obvious but very fundamental questions.

> This happened to 38-year-old Mr. Stevens, who was diagnosed with walking pneumonia. He was relieved to be sent home with a prescription for antibiotics, but completely forgot to ask important questions like, "Is the pneumonia contagious and are my family members at risk for getting the infection?" "Can I leave the house or do I need to stay at home?" "Can I go to work?" "How serious is this diagnosis?"
>
> Mr. Stevens called Dr. Stuart the next day to ask these questions but Dr. Stuart was unavailable until two days later.

Instead of conjuring up your questions during this important meeting with your doctor, come prepared to the office with a list of questions. Take Form 15 with you, ask the doctor the questions that apply to you, and fill in the answers for future reference.

Explanation of Form 15

When my doctor told me my diagnosis, I asked her how sure she was about it and whether it would be worth confirming this by getting another opinion. She seemed very offended by my comment and defensively listed her credentials. Was it wrong to ask for a second opinion?

The Accuracy of the Diagnosis

The first section of the form deals with accuracy of the diagnosis. When you ask your doctor questions in order to become confident about the diagnosis you have been given, you are not disputing the doctor's knowledge or integrity, but rather trying to better understand your illness. A request for a second opinion should never be challenged by your doctor. It is also reasonable to raise questions about information learned elsewhere that appears to contradict the doctor's conclusions, as well as to inquire about how thorough the evaluation was. So long as these questions are not asked in a hostile or challenging fashion, a competent doctor should feel comfortable expressing what is known about your diagnosis and what remains unclear.

Causes of Illness

The next section of Form 15 deals with what doctors call *etiology*, the cause of the problem. Many times, a cause cannot be determined, but there is still relief that the diagnosis has been identified and that serious illnesses, such as cancer, have been reasonably ruled out. Sometimes, etiologies cannot be identified because medical science has not advanced far enough to explain the root causes. In other cases, the causes of illness in a specific individual may not be apparent. However, even in the absence of a specific diagnosis, your doctor may still be able to offer effective treatments.

Some diagnoses tend to run in families, and this is important to know because other family members may want to be screened or, if appropriate, take preventive measures against developing the same illness you have. For example, a family member of an individual who develops heart disease may want to be especially careful about maintaining a healthy, low-fat diet and increasing exercise. Alternatively, you would want to know if an illness is contagious in order to take proper precautions.

When I met my new doctor, he seemed surprised that nobody had ever mentioned that surgery could be done to treat and possibly even cure my condition. I never imagined that surgery was an option and never thought to ask. I figured if my doctor was giving me a specific treatment, it must be the only reasonable therapy out there.

Treatment and Dealing With Illness

The subsequent section of Form 15 involves treatment. These questions are designed to acquire an overview of the medical, surgical, and other therapies appropriate for your diagnosis. More specific questions about treatment, such as how a medication is administered, drug interactions, and possible side effects are discussed in Chapter 7. Asking your doctor about the broad range of treatment options available is important, because some doctors limit their discussion only to the treatments they are familiar with. Insisting on knowing the general array of treatment options is important both at the time that diagnosis is revealed as well as during the course of treatment, especially if results are less than satisfactory.

My doctor gave me a prescription, but he did not mention whether exercise, a special diet, or anything else could be used to help my symptoms.

Beyond merely dispensing pills or performing surgery, doctors should advise you about changes in lifestyle—for example, stress reduction, stopping smoking, exercise, and diet, which can reduce the severity of a disorder or prevent a recurrence. For example, if you have high blood pressure, your doctor should advise you to stop smoking and reduce the salt in your diet.

I feel very alone with the news about my diagnosis. It would be very helpful to talk to other people who have gone through what I am going through.

Improve your knowledge about your illness and, if possible, talk to others who have also gone through this experience. The doctor may have pamphlets that elaborate on your diagnosis or be able to recommend support groups and social service agencies that can provide additional assistance and information.

Course of the Illness

The next section of Form 15 deals with prognosis or the expected course of the diagnosis. No doctor has a crystal ball. However, a doctor's accumulated knowledge drawn from his direct experience, the teachings of others, and the medical literature permits the doctor to convey a general prediction about the typical course of a disease.

When I called the doctor about a mild headache, she seemed annoyed that I was troubling her about such a minor symptom. The next week, when I developed a fever, she was mad at me for not notifying her about this new problem.

After a diagnosis is rendered, many people remain in a quandary as to when they should notify the doctor about new or recurrent symptoms. Some people neglect to call the doctor even in the face of very significant symptoms out of fear of bothering the doctor. While discretion should be used, you do not do the doctor or yourself a favor by being considerate if the end-result is a major complication from delayed attention to a problem. To address this concern, it is helpful at the outset to clarify with the doctor when it is appropriate to call with an urgent question or problem, when you can wait till regular office hours, and when to go to the emergency room. Discussing this in advance will allow you to feel more comfortable when calling and the doctor more concerned when your call is received.

How Will the Diagnosis Affect My Life?

The most neglected area relating to a diagnosis concerns the psychosocial implications. By this we mean the way the illness affects diverse aspects of your life, such as home life, studies, relationships, travel, exercise, recreation, and work. Recently, and unfortunately belatedly, medical science has finally begun to recognize the importance of focusing not only on treating symptoms but also trying to improve the quality of life of those in their care. Discussing the effects of illness on the many facets of our lives is the first step toward finding ways to maintain or enhance the quality of life in the face of illness.

MEDICAL ECONOMICS

Second Opinions

> "In cases where there is trouble making a diagnosis, I make sure the patient knows that I truly care about what is happening, that I believe they have something real, and that I will do everything I can. I will take whatever information is available, and I will collaborate. In this case the parents came up with some information that was very important. They were better doctors than me. But what I was able to do was remain open-minded so that I could help them better. If I had ignored what they were discovering I would not have been a very good doctor at all. I am not here to be right. I am not here to be the god of medicine. I am here to help."
>
> MIKE MAGEE AND MICHAEL D'ANTONIO
> *Good Karma: The Best Medicine*

There are times when a definitive diagnosis cannot be achieved, despite a doctor's best efforts. Lack of a diagnosis can be very unsettling, and the comfort levels of doctor and patient in this situation can be very different. (Ask your doctor if she has considered the causes for commonly encountered symptoms by referring to Appendix C.) In the absence of a firm diagnosis, some people may be relieved that serious conditions have been ruled out. Others worry that this means a serious illness is still lurking, waiting to cause them further medical problems at a later date. Sometimes, the unsettling feeling is so intense that it feels better having a bad diagnosis than no diagnosis at all. These are all commonly encountered reactions.

There are several possible explanations for an inability to make a diagnosis. The least likely possibility is that an unusual, new kind of disease has developed. More likely is the possibility that your doctor does not deal with your particular medical problem on a regular basis and is unfamiliar with the nuances of your case. Indeed, with the explosion of advances in medicine, it becomes increasingly difficult for doctors to stay on top of so many different areas of medical science. Alternatively, the doctor may be pursuing incorrect diagnostic reasoning or have failed to recognize some crucial findings. Regardless, when the diagnosis is unclear, it is very appropriate to get additional opinions. Many fine doctors will spontaneously suggest getting another opinion and may provide names of experts that deal with your particular problem. Doctors who do so should not be viewed as conceding defeat or displaying lack of ability; rather, these are responsible doctors who consider your health to be a top priority. If your doctor does not suggest a second opinion, it is appropriate to ask about it.

If you are at odds with your doctor about your diagnosis or treatment options, it may be advisable to get names of other doctors to contact for a second opinion from other sources, because a doctor recommended by your primary doctor may not be inclined to openly disagree with a friend or close colleague. Here is an example where even the authors fell victim to a doctor's discouraging a vitally needed second opinion:

> A 70-year-old relative of ours was hospitalized for chest pain and scheduled for angioplasty (a procedure to widen the arteries supplying the heart). While one of us was on the phone strongly urging her to get a second opinion, her cardiologist walked into her room and overheard the conversation. He told her that her problem was clear-cut and that she did not need a second opinion. She followed the doctor's advice, underwent an angioplasty, and was discharged three days later. The following day, she returned to the hospital with a massive heart attack. Several weeks later, another cardiologist reviewed the coronary artery films that were taken preceding the angioplasty and indicated that if he had managed her case, he would never have

attempted to correct such extensive and widespread blood vessel narrowings with angioplasty; he would have rushed her for coronary artery bypass surgery. She and her family now have to live with the aftermath of this devastating complication.

Don't Worry; It's All in Your Head!

Second opinions are not only helpful when a diagnosis is unclear, but sometimes they should be considered even when a diagnosis is rendered—for example, when major decisions hinge on an accurate diagnosis or when symptoms persist despite recommended treatment. Second opinions are also appropriate when symptoms are dismissed as purely psychological in nature, especially if the diagnosis is given in the absence of reasonable testing. The medical literature is filled with terrible stories of missed diagnoses attributed to purely psychological causes. Although there are indeed psychologically-driven symptoms, this conclusion should be made only with great caution and after very careful evaluation.

Your Doctor Should Welcome a Second Opinion

A second opinion can give fresh insights or further clarify the diagnosis, lead to a different diagnosis, or arrive at similar conclusions about the diagnosis. It can also include suggestions for other treatments. Rather than a statement of poor confidence in the original doctor, second opinions should be welcomed by patient and doctor alike in order to help both of them deal with medical symptoms. For example, second opinions may reinforce confidence in the recommendations of the first doctor. Sometimes, an arrangement can be made between doctors wherein the primary doctor manages the day-to-day problems but confers with the specialist as needed when specific difficulties arise. This is gratifying for both of the doctors and comforting for the patient. It is unfortunate when doctors view the idea of another medical opinion with severe hostility. Refusal to confer with another doctor does a great disservice to everyone.

Questions to Ask About Your Diagnosis

Accuracy of Diagnosis

What is the diagnosis? _____

_____

_____

If a diagnosis has not been determined, what serious diseases have been
ruled out? Could I still have something serious? _____

_____

_____

How confident is the doctor about the accuracy of the diagnosis? _____

_____

_____

Could it be something else? _____

_____

_____

How did the doctor arrive at this specific diagnosis? _____

_____

_____

Are any other tests or consultations with specialists indicated? _____

_____

_____

Causes of Illness

What caused this illness? How did I get it? _____

_____

_____

Does this illness run in families? _____

Is it contagious? _____

Treatment and Dealing with Your Illness

How is this illness treated? Are medications, surgery, or other treatments recommended? _____

_____

_____

Can a change in lifestyle or diet reduce the severity of the disease or combat the illness? _____

_____

_____

Are there pamphlets, books, or other forms of information that the doctor can provide? _____

_____

_____

Are there any organizations that can offer additional information or support? _____

_____

_____

What medical follow-up should I get and how often? _____

_____

_____

Course of the Illness

What is the usual course or prognosis of this illness? Is it progressive? Life-threatening? _____

_____

_____

What parts of the body does this illness affect now and in the future? Is it associated with other complications? _____

_____

_____

Will it affect my ability to have children? _____

_____

Will it cause any cosmetic or disfiguring effects? _____

_____

_____

What further symptoms or problems should I look out for, and when
should I notify others or my doctor about them? _____

_____

_____

How Will the Diagnosis Affect My Life?

Ask your doctor how your illness will affect you in the following areas:

Home life _____

Work _____

Studies _____

Relationships _____

Exercise and recreational activities _____

Travel _____

CHAPTER 21

If You Do not Ask Questions About Your Medications, You are Asking for Trouble

"My medical team bombarded me with facts, statistics, and survival rates. One cell. More than three positive lymph nodes involved. If I did not take chemotherapy, there was a 75 percent chance of recurrence, and I would have a 25 percent chance of survival. If I did take the chemotherapy, I would reduce the chances of recurrence by 75 percent.

Here were these men, my friends as well as my doctors, telling me facts crucial to my making decisions about my life and death. I could not hear them. I sat calmly while they talked, giving every outward appearance of attention, but I blotted out everything they said. I did not hear their voices. I did not see their faces. Their facts did not apply to me. I had too many things to do, too much life left to live."

RENA BLUMBERG
Headstrong: A Story of Conquests and Celebrations…
Living Through Chemotherapy

You have been very diligent! You prepared detailed information about your symptoms and helped your doctor arrive at a diagnosis. But preparing for your next visit to the doctor does not stop there. Now it is time to consider treatment. Form 16 provides a list of questions that you can ask your doctor about treatment.

My doctor prescribed a drug, but the brand-name version is very expensive. Is a cheaper generic version just as good as the brand-name drug?

Medications are identified by a generic and a brand-name; it is useful to be familiar with both names. The generic name is the identification of the drug that remains the same irrespective of the manufacturer; it is the nonproprietary name that is not protected by a trademark. The brand-name is the name given to a drug by the manufacturer. If the same medication is manufactured by different companies, each company gives it a different brand-name. (The brand and generic names of commonly prescribed medications are listed in Appendix D, along with questions you can ask your doctor about the specific drugs you are receiving.)

Brand-name versions of a drug tend to be more expensive than generic versions. In the first few years after the introduction of a drug, the drug is under patent and independent generic versions of the drug are not available. Generic forms of the drug may become available at a later date. It is useful to inquire about the cost of the drug, particularly if you do not have insurance to cover the cost of an expensive medication and it is going to be taken for a prolonged period of time. Why not simply insist on receiving the generic form if it is cheaper? One reason is that some brand-name drugs may have superior characteristics compared to generic drugs. Another problem is that a given disorder may need strict consistency in the percentage of the drug absorbed into the body and in other drug-related characteristics. Even if the generic drug is not inferior to the brand-name, many manufacturers produce different generic forms of the drug and there is no way to guarantee that you will receive the exact same generic formulation each time the prescription is filled. This creates problems because the drugs may not be exactly alike and levels in the bloodstream may vary.

I just left the doctor's office with my new prescription. Then I realized that I do not know whether I should take the last dose in the afternoon or at night before going to sleep.

Learning the right way to take a medication is essential to achieving the full effectiveness of that medication and reducing your chances of incurring undesired effects. Insist that your doctor carefully explain how the medication should be taken. Learning about your diagnosis and treatment recommendations in the short amount of time allotted for office visits can make it difficult to quickly digest important information. It is helpful to have the doctor write out the dosage of each pill, how many pills should be taken, and at what time of day. This is especially crucial if the medication is being started at one particular dose, but the dose may be changed in the future. Some medications are administered with pamphlets or instruction cards for proper use. Take Form 16 with you to the doctor's office, ask the questions that pertain to your medical situation, and fill in the doctor's answers for future reference.

It is helpful to learn about the typical range of dosing customarily used for your medication and how high you can anticipate going if necessary in the future. Knowing this information in advance will help you understand whether the drug is likely to be abandoned if it does not work or, instead, advanced in dosage in the hope that a higher dose will achieve the desired effect.

Drug Absorption

A pill or capsule has to dissolve in the juices of the stomach after it is swallowed and be absorbed into the body before it can have an effect. Most of the medication is then absorbed further down in the lining of the small intestine. The degree and rate of drug absorption is dependent on many conditions, including the chemical makeup of the drug, the dosage, how it is given, interactions with other medications and contents in the stomach, and specific aspects of a person's health. Medications administered in fluid form rather than hard pills may have faster but not necessarily better absorption. Medication coating, often included to reduce gastrointestinal irritation, can also interfere with absorption. Medication that is injected into the muscle has to be absorbed into the bloodstream.[10]

Taking some medications at the same time as another medication can potentially drastically change the level of the second medication in the bloodstream. Some drugs are best taken on an empty stomach in order to avoid being inactivated or have interference with drug absorption; others are more appropriately taken during or after a meal in order to reduce stomach irritation or side effects from the drug being absorbed too quickly. This needs to be clarified with the doctor.

Some people, particularly children or individuals with medical conditions, may have difficulty swallowing a pill whole and might prefer chewing or crushing the pill and mixing it with food. While this may create no problems for some medications, others should never be crushed or chewed. Some drugs can be administered with food; others have their absorption disturbed by food. Some medications can be given in a liquid solution. However, even if the dosage administered is exactly the same as the pill dosage, absorption of the drug may be different and the total dose prescribed may need to be changed.

Storing Medicines

Ms. Brannigan is a 70-year-old woman with recurring angina, chest pain due to blockage of the blood vessels supplying the heart. Usually, her chest pain goes away promptly after placing a nitroglycerin tablet under her tongue. Her typical chest pain started one day while she was shopping, but this time it did not get better even after taking two nitroglycerin tablets. She went to the emergency room and was very concerned that her unrelenting chest pain meant she was having a heart attack. She was given nitroglycerin in the emergency room and her pain went away immediately. Fortunately, there was no evidence of a heart attack.

When reviewing her medications with the doctor, she showed him her jar of nitroglycerin tablets. Upon examination,

10. *Nursing 2001 Drug Handbook.* Springhouse, Pa.: Springhouse Corporation, 2001.

the doctor discovered that the nitroglycerin had exceeded its expiration date. In retrospect, Ms. Brannigan realized that she had been carrying around an old jar of ineffective pills.

Some medications need to be stored in a particular fashion—for example, in a dark cabinet or at certain temperatures. Pharmacists are often very helpful resources to clarify such information. Medications should be kept in their original bottles in locations that are not accessible to children. *Never* take a medication prescribed for someone else. Check the drug container labels for expiration dates and replace the drug with a fresh supply if the date has exceeded the expiration time. Avoid storing medications in your bathroom because of the significant humidity in that environment.

I forgot to take my pill and got very worried my infection would get worse. So I decided to take an extra pill later in the day. Then I worried whether I did the right thing. What should I have done?

The more times a drug needs to be taken during the day, the higher the chance of forgetting a dose. All of us forget to take our medicines once in a while. Ask your doctor if this would cause a particularly serious problem with your medication and how to handle the situation should you forget a dose. Alternatively, if you mistakenly take too much in one day, ask your doctor how dangerous this might be.

The Body's Garbage Disposal System

Another consideration in dosing a medication has to do with *distribution*. A drug is absorbed and then distributed to various parts of the body. The doctor needs to adjust some medication dosages to accommodate changes in the way the medication is distributed due to the changes in fluid that occur with generalized body swelling conditions or loss of fluid from dehydration. Some medications are not well distributed into the fatty tissues of the body. If dosing is based only on weight, which may increase due to an increase in body fat, and your doctor ends up giving you too much of a drug, you may be at risk for experiencing toxic side effects.[11] The body rids itself of medication by excreting (removing) the drug through the kidneys, the liver, and in more rare circumstances, through other parts of the body. In a process called *metabolism*, many drugs undergo a process of change in structure to become more inactive substances. Metabolism usually occurs in the liver. The rate of metabolism can vary greatly from one individual to another. This leads to differences in drug blood levels. Your doctor may test your blood level to decide whether a dosage adjustment is needed. Drug levels may drop too low if your

11. *Nursing 2001 Drug Handbook.* Springhouse, Pa.: Springhouse Corporation, 2001.

metabolic rate is too high, and routine doses can cause toxic effects if your metabolic rate is too low.

Diseases of the liver can change the degree and rate of metabolism. Most of the time, liver disease results in reduced metabolism, thereby raising the risk of causing elevations in drug levels, sometimes to toxic amounts.

The small decreases in kidney function that occur as we grow older reduce the rate of elimination of drugs in the body, resulting in higher blood levels and a lower dose requirement, or a reduction in the number of times the drug is taken during the day. Doctors sometimes forget to make these adjustments. Diseases of the kidneys can result in significant problems in excreting drugs or their metabolized drug forms (*metabolites*). In severe kidney disease, drugs and other toxins accumulating in the body can be removed with a procedure called *dialysis*.

In summary, if you have liver or kidney problems, ask your doctor if the doses of your medications have been adjusted accordingly.

Medication Travels

Drugs are carried throughout the body on proteins circulating in the blood. The active portion of a drug is the portion that is released from the protein so it can act on different parts of the body. Conditions that lower levels of protein, such as malnutrition or being elderly, can lead to higher unbound portions of drug, which may result in side-effects due to the excess of drug. Similarly, adding other drugs that compete with the first drug for binding with proteins can bump off the first drug from these chemical carriers, resulting in toxic effects. Ask your doctor whether he considered these possible drug interactions when he prescribed your drug dosage.

Duration of Treatment

Ask your doctor how long he intends to administer your treatment. Decisions about the duration of treatment are based on many factors, including the nature of the disorder, the purpose of the treatment, and whether the disorder is considered to be a temporary condition or a long-term problem. Asking about the duration of your intended treatment will help you understand more about your diagnosis and prognosis.

My doctor saw me quickly and sent me out with a prescription. I wonder whether the drug he prescribed is the only treatment that works. What other choices are there?

In an age when more active partnership in decision-making is promoted in the doctor-patient relationship, questions about effectiveness and side effects of drug should be asked without reservation. Such questions include: "How does the drug work?" and "What is the purpose of using this treatment?" Is the intent to cure the problem, control symptoms completely without curing the problem, or merely reduce the severity of symptoms? Surprisingly, most medications are prescribed to control symptoms rather than completely cure a medical condition. In life, everything we do has risks and benefits. Our decision to get into a car and travel to the supermarket is based on our weighing the benefits of obtaining groceries over the remote risk of getting into a car accident. In a similar way, the doctor's decision to prescribe a medication is based on a decision that the potential benefits of the drug outweigh the possible risks. Discussion of the risks and benefits of any intervention, surgical or medical, has become the standard of care, and you should insist on discussing this. Sometimes, side effects of a medication are so severe and the benefits so weak, that abstaining from treatment may be a very appropriate decision. For example, in the face of some severe malignancies, specific chemotherapeutic agents may not have proven effectiveness and yet may be frequently associated with severe side effects that could greatly compromise quality of life.

It is helpful to know whether your doctor believes the prescribed medication is the only one available to treat your condition—this is rarely the case—or whether other options are available. If so, why did your doctor select this particular drug? Selection of a treatment should be based on many factors, including the drug's effectiveness, how well it is tolerated, how easy it is to administer, the cost, whether there are drug interactions, and other features. Sometimes a drug is selected because it coincidentally treats more than one of the conditions that you are experiencing. Unfortunately, doctors sometimes prescribe the drug they are simply the most comfortable with, perhaps having learned to use one drug during their training and having little experience with newer compounds. People should inquire about other treatments, including those that may not be available through their doctor.

Does use of a medication follow established guidelines? Is it FDA-approved for the condition being treated? If not, why is the doctor prescribing the drug in this way? Further, how much experience has been acquired with this drug? A drug undergoes extensive testing in sequential phases before it comes to market, beginning with animal studies, followed by administration to healthy volunteers, and then testing in individuals with a specific medical condition. While this degree of testing should be reassuring as to the issue of serious side effects, in fact, many surprises about a drug emerge after it is dispensed more widely in general clinical practice. For one thing, the number of people exposed to a drug that it takes to uncover uncommon side effects far surpasses the typical number of individuals tested in pre-marketing studies.

Additionally, pre-marketing studies are artificial, experimental conditions in which fixed doses are used. They may not represent how the drug will end up being used in the real world. Pre-marketing trials usually last for only short periods of time and therefore give little insight into long-term effects. Subtle kinds of side effects, such as change in mood, are often under-reported during pre-marketing drug trials. On the other hand, because of the way questions are asked during pre-marketing trials, some side effects are over-emphasized and potentially good effects other than the main endpoint of the study are often missed. Certain drug combinations may also not be tested in pre-marketing investigations, and we may only subsequently learn about dangers when mixing the medication with other drugs.

Side Effects

It seems fundamental; yet, countless doctors prescribe drugs without informing their patients about potential side effects. If you encounter this situation, it is appropriate to insist on reviewing this crucial information. One of the best ways to convey this information is for the doctor to provide written materials and then highlight the main effects. Information specifically written for the layman is generally superior to the laundry list of information from the *Physician's Desk Reference* (PDR), because the latter uses more difficult-to-understand medical terminology and lists virtually any effects that were experienced during pre-marketing studies, which may have been coincidental symptoms rather than direct effects of the drug.

Medication side effects may be categorized as either *idiosyncratic* or *dose-related*. Idiosyncratic effects are side effects that occur irrespective of the amount of drug used. Fortunately, they are usually rare, though they can be serious. We do not know why one individual gets this type of side effect while another does not, but we speculate that some individuals have a genetic susceptibility to certain drug reactions. Examples of idiosyncratic reactions include allergic reactions, acute hepatitis (resulting in liver inflammation), and interference with the production of blood cells from bone marrow. Idiosyncratic effects are therefore not resolved by reducing the dose. In such cases, it is unclear whether frequent blood testing will catch such a reaction early enough before it becomes serious. Nevertheless, your doctor will likely order blood tests on occasion if there is a risk of idiosyncratic effects. Reporting any unusual symptoms immediately to your doctor is perhaps more effective than blood test screening. Fortunately, most idiosyncratic side effects occur only within the first few weeks to months of drug use.

Dose-related side effects, on the other hand, occur after increasing the dose of a medication and tend to get worse as the dose is further advanced. In the event of a dose-related side effect, the side effects may improve spontaneously with time; they may respond to slight dose reduction; they may have to be endured because the drug benefit is so important and no alternative treatments are available; or they may warrant discontinuation of the drug. Some drug side effects are not easily classified as idiosyncratic or dose-related.

Sometimes the body gets used to a drug that it did not tolerate well when it was first introduced. It is important for doctors and patients not to immediately abandon a drug if this occurs, because in the long term it may be a potentially highly effective and well-tolerated treatment. Hastily discontinuing a drug every time there is even a mild side effect can lead to there being no options left for treatment. Drugs are introduced at the doses used in pre-marketing studies, but experience often leads to starting treatment at a lower dose with more gradual advancement over time in order to improve tolerance of the drug.

It is important to know what should be done in the event of a side effect. When should the doctor be notified? Should any precautions be taken if a drug is known to cause possible side effects? For example, ask your doctor if driving is inadvisable because of anticipated drug-induced drowsiness, or whether exposure to the sun should be limited because the drug causes sensitivity to light.

My doctor keeps checking the level of the medication in my bloodstream. Why does she do this? What is she looking for?

Measuring drug levels can provide evidence of suspected excess of a drug in a person's system. However, everyone has their own unique tolerance levels and their own level needed for drug effectiveness. An acceptable dosage in one individual may be poorly tolerated in another. A classic example is in the elderly, in which dose-related side effects may occur in spite of drug levels in the purported acceptable range. Therefore, drug levels should be used only as a rough guide for dosing medication. Doctors do best by treating the person, rather than treating with standard levels.

Another way to look at side effects is according to when they occur. Short-term effects refers to those side effects that occur immediately or days to weeks after the introduction of a new medication. Long-term side effects may mean effects that occur after weeks to months on a drug, but usually this means years of medication use. Acute allergic reactions or nausea in response to taking a pill are examples of short-term side effects. Examples of long-term effects include cumulative effects on the liver or developing fragile bones (osteoporosis).

Side effects may also be classified according to the part of the body affected —for example:

Skin Rash

I began itching after I started the new medication. Is this an emergency or should I wait till my next appointment with the doctor?

Some medications may cause allergic reactions. While most rashes caught in their earliest phases will resolve easily with the discontinuation of the drug, some can progress to very serious and, rarely, life-threatening forms of rash. Your doctor should be notified at the first sign of a rash. In some cases, the rash may be caused by other factors unrelated to the drug, and the doctor may recommend continuing the medication. This decision should be based on, at a minimum, a telephone conversation and more ideally by prompt evaluation in the office. If a rash is progressing and the doctor has not observed the rash, it is appropriate to insist on being seen immediately, even if this requires a visit to the emergency room. Most allergic reactions to drugs occur within the first weeks to months after starting a drug. On the other hand, it is very uncommon for allergic reactions to develop after many years of taking a medicine.

Drop in Blood Counts

Some medications can cause lowering of red and white blood cell or platelet counts. Mild reductions in blood counts may be completely acceptable and result in no problems for the body's normal functioning. More severe reductions can cause significant anemia, higher risk of infection, and a tendency toward bleeding (respectively). If a drug is known to carry risks of blood count abnormalities, it is traditional to undergo repeat blood testing to check for these abnormalities. However, the usefulness of frequent, intermittent blood testing to screen for the most serious forms of blood count abnormalities is controversial, because even if a serious abnormality occurs, testing the blood every day may not prevent it from progressing once it has happened. Fortunately, for many drugs, the most serious forms of drop in blood count tend to occur within the first year of using the drug, and the chances become very slim after many years of drug usage.

Liver

I heard that the drug I receive can cause liver damage, so I was really surprised when my doctor did not seem to care that a few of my liver function tests were slightly elevated.

The liver is the metabolic engine of the body, and it can be affected by many kinds of drugs. Sometimes, blood tests measuring liver function can be mildly abnormal without signifying a significant liver problem. This is because drugs that are metabolized in the liver may cause some of the normal liver enzymes to spill out into the blood without causing a specific liver injury. Alternatively, toxicity of the liver can be very serious and liver functions are typically included in screening blood tests to exclude this possibility. In people with a history of liver disease or risk of liver disease, such as those with alcoholism, the doctor may select a drug to use that will not affect, and will not be affected by the liver.

Gastrointestinal System

Some drugs cause irritation of the stomach and intestines, leading to abdominal pain or nausea. Less commonly, abdominal pain can be a sign of serious illness of the gastrointestinal system. It is important to clarify how urgently the doctor should be notified in the event of abdominal symptoms and what can be done to rectify the problem if it occurs.

Birth Defects

My doctor told me I need to get off some of my medications because they are listed as "Category C." What does this mean?

Some drugs carry a risk of inducing birth defects when taken during pregnancy. Frequently, it is difficult to get a specific handle on the exact risks of a given medication because it takes rigorous study of very large numbers of exposed individuals to estimate risk. Animal studies can be helpful, but safety in animals does not necessarily translate into safety in humans. Medications are classified into broad categories of estimated risk of inducing birth defects. *Category A* refers to the safest drugs, with no evidence of harm to the baby. *Category B* suggests slightly higher risk (animal studies safe but no human data, or animal studies show a risk). *Category C* means animal studies show a risk but there is no information on humans, or there is no information in either animals or humans. *Category D* means there is evidence of risk to humans but benefits may still outweigh the risks. *Category X* means strong evidence, and animal and human studies suggest that the drug should absolutely not be used when pregnant.[12]

Learning that you are pregnant while on a risky drug usually means that the baby has been exposed to the drug for at least a few weeks. The most crucial period for drug-induced abnormalities in development of the baby occurs during the first trimester of pregnancy. Therefore, it is best to consider the risk of birth defects even before getting pregnant so that the safest regimen can be prescribed ahead of time. Some birth defects are prevented by taking daily folic acid, although it is unclear if this includes drug-induced birth defects. Taking the smallest number of different medications at the lowest reasonable dose is the safest strategy if drugs must be taken during pregnancy.

12. *Drugs in Pregnancy and Lactation* by G.G. Briggs, R.K. Freeman, and S.J. Yaffe. Baltimore: Williams & Wilkins, 1998. Page XXII.

Brain

Many drugs have effects on the brain, causing fatigue, sleepiness or difficulty sleeping, mood changes, dizziness, headache, and tremors. These side effects can be easily glossed over during a medical evaluation. While doctors may think you are doing great because the drug is working, you may actually feel terrible, experience a lack of energy, and have the need to nap all the time. You need to let your doctor know if this is the case.

Heart and Vascular System

Some medications cause undesirable effects on the heart, such as irregular heart beats, and on the blood vessel (vascular) system, such as a significant drop in blood pressure. Discuss the potential risks with your doctor and how you can be on guard for these problems.

Hormones and Sexuality

Some drugs cause changes in hormone levels, which in turn create problems in normal body function. Discussion of sexual dysfunction is often neglected in doctor-patient encounters. In some cases, this is due to medication revving up the liver and lowering the levels of testosterone, a hormone that is essential for normal sexual response and performance. (Hormones are also discussed in Chapter 12.)

Kidneys

My doctor was completely unaware that I have a history of kidney stones. Fortunately, I insisted that he review the main side effects of the new drug he planned to prescribe. When he mentioned kidney stones, I reminded him about my prior kidney problem and he decided not to prescribe the drug after all!

The effects of drugs on the kidneys include inducing kidney stones, impairing kidney function, or otherwise injuring the kidney. Make sure your doctor knows about any prior history of kidney stones, having only one kidney, or a family history of kidney problems.

Increasing the Risk of Developing Cancer

Based on animal studies, some drugs are believed to be associated with an elevated risk of developing cancer. However, there are theoretical limitations in generalizing effects from animal studies and applying them to humans. Studies of humans are limited by the extraordinarily large number of exposures needed to generate an idea about risk of cancer. Therefore, medical science is often unsure about the distinct risk of cancer with specific drugs.

Immune Reactions

Inflammatory reactions, such as autoimmunity, in which the body is tricked into attacking itself, are occasionally provoked by medication. For example, some drugs are said to cause reactions similar to lupus or blood vessel inflammations called *vasculitis*. (Lupus is an autoimmune illness affecting many parts of the body.)

Drug Interactions

Keep in mind that some medications significantly interact with prescribed medications, nonprescription agents, or foods. Use of alcohol may also be inadvisable when taking certain medications.

Special Situations

Sometimes, doctors are so focused on your current medical problems they forget your history of allergic reactions or other medical conditions that make a new medication risky to use. Remind your doctor if this is the case.

Medications may contain ingredients, such as salt or sugar, which may be suboptimal for use by some people—for example, people who have high blood pressure or diabetes, respectively. Risks associated with drugs during pregnancy have been discussed earlier. However, risk to babies from medication transmitted via breast milk varies depending on the specific drug and should be discussed as well. Traces of most medications can be found in breast milk, with the highest levels occurring soon after taking the dose. Therefore, it is usually advisable to breastfeed before taking a medication rather than after.

Finally, to understand the long-term strategy of treating medical problems, doctor and patient can begin looking ahead to future options should the present treatment fail to work or is poorly tolerated.

Medication Questions

Name of drug:

What is the name of the medication (both generic and brand-name)? _____

_____

Does it matter whether the generic or brand-name drug is taken? _____

_____

How costly is the drug? _____

Proper Way to Take the Medication:

What is the proper way to take the medication? _____

_____

What is the specific dosage? _____

What is the typical dosage range and how high can the dose be raised? ____

_____

When should each dose be taken? _____

_____

Are there any foods, drinks, or other medicines (prescription and
nonprescription) that should be avoided when taking this medication? _____

_____

_____

Should it be taken with food or on an empty stomach? _____

Should it be taken whole, or can it be crushed or chewed before swallowing?

_____

What should be done if a dose is missed? What should be done if too much
is taken? _____

_____

How long will I be on the drug? _____

Does the drug need to be stored in any special way? _____

_____

Drug Effects:

How does the drug work? _____

_____

How effective is the drug? Will it cure my problem? If not, what benefits will it bring? _____

_____

_____

Is not taking medicine an option? Do the benefits of taking it outweigh the risks? _____

_____

_____

Are there alternatives to this medication? Why was this medication selected over others? _____

_____

_____

Is this drug a standard FDA-approved treatment or is it experimental? Does it follow any standardized treatment guidelines? _____

_____

How long has this drug been on the market? _____

How will I feel on the drug? _____

_____

Are there any side effects (short-term vs. long-term, rare or unexpected vs. dose-related)? _____

_____

Will it affect the ability to have sex? _____

_____

What symptoms or side effects should I be on the alert for? _____

_____

What should I do if side effects occur? How long do they usually last? _____

_____

Do I need to call the doctor if I experience a given side effect? _____

_____

Does the medication require any monitoring, such as blood tests? _____

_____

Are there any restrictions in activities while taking this medication, such as driving or exposure to the sun? _____ `

_____

Drug Interactions:

Is this drug safe to take with my other medications? _____

_____

Can I take it at the same time as I take other medications (prescription or non-prescription)? _____

_____

Can I drink alcohol while I am taking the medication? _____

Special Situations:

Are there any problems taking this medication in light of my other medical problems? _____

_____

If there is a history of allergies to any medicine, foods, dyes, or other ingredients: Is there a risk of an allergic reaction to this medication? _____

_____

If on a special diet: Does the medication contain an excess amount of a substance I should not take, such as salt or sugar? _____

_____

If currently or planning to become pregnant: Are there risks in taking this medication during pregnancy? _____

_____

If currently or planning to breastfeed: Are there any risks to the baby from my taking this drug during breastfeeding? _____

_____

Future Plans:

What are my options if this treatment does not work? _____

_____

_____

CHAPTER 22

Surgery and Other Procedures Are Not a Cut and Dry Matter

"Before he operates, the surgeon must believe that the patient will be better off because of his efforts, and his self-confidence has to border on bravado if he is to pick up a knife and start cutting. Here both training and judgment are paramount. Knowing when not to operate is just as important as operating.

In most cases the surgeon has a definite procedure in mind before attempting an operation, but occasionally an unexpected, alarming condition is uncovered that changes everything. Many times when scrubbing before surgery I have paused briefly to ask the Lord not to desert me in my efforts."

HULL COOK
50 Years a Country Doctor

"You need surgery!" These words can be very frightening. How can you best prepare to ask the important questions in the midst of this anxiety? Using Form 17 is one way to focus on the questions you need to ask your primary doctor and the surgeon who will perform the procedure. The questions on this form are applicable for outpatient surgical procedures as well as inpatient hospitalizations. Take Form 17 with you to your pre-surgical meeting with your doctors, ask the questions that apply to your situation, and record the answers so you can read them at home and make sure you understand them.

The Risks of Surgery

Doctors are taught to discuss the risks and benefits of any procedure with their patients and document in the medical record that this information was conveyed. Unfortunately, this is not always done or if it is done, it may not necessarily cover the important issues thoroughly. Therefore, you need to take an active approach and insist on understanding the nature of the surgery, even if your doctor seems pressed for time. Many surgeries carry substantial risk of complications, even the risk of dying. This is a tough subject to discuss, but it has to be faced head on. You are entitled to know how often complications occur and what measures are taken to avoid these complications.

Your Surgeon's Qualifications

Many people are too inhibited to ask their surgeon about his qualifications and ability to perform the recommended surgery. On the other hand, when you hire a painter or plumber to work on your house, it is customary to get information about the person who will do the work rather than hiring a perfect stranger. Why do less when it comes to your health care?

Beyond questioning your surgeon directly, some of this information may be available in medical specialty books at the library or on the Internet. Sometimes, it is easier to inquire about a surgeon's qualifications by asking your primary care doctor.

As discussed in Chapter 20, consider getting a second opinion. This does not need to be perceived as a threat to your primary doctor's integrity and, in fact, it may reinforce confidence in the approach taken by the surgeon. Many insurance companies will subsidize a second opinion and may even encourage it.

Before the Surgery Is Performed

What preparations will be needed before the surgery and what restrictions or precautions should you know about before the surgery? For example, can you take aspirin, which promotes a tendency to bleed, before the surgery? What should be done about daily warfarin (Coumadin®) dosing before surgery? Are there any restrictions on eating before the surgery? Asking questions such as these in advance can help prevent possible complications.

The Surgery

They sent a resident doctor to see me before the surgery. I asked him if my doctor was going to perform the surgery or whether he would be doing it. He became angry with me for asking, so I asked to speak to my own doctor. Unfortunately, he was unavailable, and I ended up going into surgery without feeling comfortable about the surgery or the surgeon. I wish I had clarified this question in advance.

Many medical centers employ junior doctors in training (residents and fellows) who assist surgeons during surgical procedures. It is perfectly appropriate to ask how much and what parts of the surgery will be performed by the training doctors and what will be performed by the attending doctor.

Find out what is actually going to be done during the surgery. Some doctors explain procedures by showing patients a diagram that highlights the body parts involved and how they will be altered during surgery. As indicated on Form 17, ask if there are different ways of doing the surgery and, if so, what are the risks and benefits of each approach? Why is one approach preferred over another? Is it because the surgeon is capable of only one approach or that the medical center is not equipped to perform other types of surgeries?

Anesthesia

Risks associated with any method of anesthesia should be discussed with the anesthesiologist directly.

- General anesthesia involves putting a person to sleep for the duration of surgery, during which breathing is controlled by a respirator and anesthetic gases are inhaled.

- Regional anesthesia entails numbing the sensation in a large portion of the body, such as an arm or leg, without putting the person to sleep. It may involve injecting an anesthetic agent into the fluid that surrounds the spine (spinal anesthesia) or the space around the spinal cord called the epidural space (epidural anesthesia).

- Local anesthesia involves injection of a numbing medication, such as lidocaine, into the body tissue where surgery will be performed. The numbing effects of the medication tend to go away after a short period of time following the surgery.

Blood Transfusions

During the surgery, you may require a transfusion to replace lost blood. You should inquire in advance about potential complications from transfusions, including the risk of developing immune reactions or infections. Sometimes, you can donate your own blood before surgery in what is called *autologous* donation. Alternatively, there may be options to use blood donated by family or friends, although studies have shown that these donations do not tend to be safer than those from healthy community volunteers. Ask your doctor if there are alternatives to having a transfusion during the surgery.

Recovery from Surgery and Pain Management

When I got out of surgery, I was in terrible pain. I called the nurses for pain medicine, but it took a very long time to reach the doctor and get an order into the chart!

> "'Is the procedure, ah, painful?' I asked, conscious of sounding like a layman again — worse still, a timorous one. I could not help it. Somehow, I felt that if I knew there was going to be pain, I could prepare myself for what was inevitably going to happen in a few moments — unless, that is, I removed the ultrasound probe, stood up, and walked out, a fantasy that occupied my mind for a second or two.
>
> He chuckled. 'Painful?' he said. 'Not for me.'
>
> He inserted the probe. 'You'll hear a click each time I pull the trigger,' he said. 'There'll be a pulling sensation, then a quick pinch — nothing to be excited about at all.'

I heard the click and felt a quick stab, followed by shame at my own cowardice.

'There,' he said cheerfully. 'I told you it was nothing. It'll be a lot easier if you just relax.'

I nodded. Relax? How, I asked myself, was I to relax while lying on my side, vulnerable and half-naked, while a doctor probed deep into my prostate, snipping off tiny plugs of tissue as a gardener might cut flowers?… I wondered why the procedure was done without Valium or any form of anesthetic, and was later (too late, alas) informed that some doctors do give their patients something to relax them before the procedure. Knowing this, I strongly recommend your asking for it — insisting on it, even — should you ever find yourself in this situation."

M. KORDA
Man to Man: Surviving Prostate Cancer

Many doctors are poorly trained in the administration of pain medications and notoriously prescribe inadequate doses. Some are inappropriately obsessed with the idea that giving a high dose of pain medication while the patient is in the hospital can lead to chronic addiction.

Depending on the type of surgery and the health of the individual, the nature and time required for recovery from surgery will vary greatly. Knowing what to expect can prepare you psychologically and give you time to arrange for people to help you or obtain home equipment. Pain is a common complication of surgery, and it is often reassuring to learn ahead of time what measures will be available to control it. Nowadays, instead of getting a pain pill or a shot at specific times ordered by the doctor, patient-controlled analgesia (pain medication; *PCA*) is often available. PCA is run through an intravenous line attached to a pump that allows you — within reasonable limits — to control the amount of painkiller you receive at any time. Instead of waiting for the doctor to be called for additional pain medication, the person can push a button and get additional medication as needed within a given range. Insist that the nurses regularly page the doctor in order to get the pain medication order written as quickly as possible if PCA is not being used.

Find out for how long after surgery you will be restricted from your regular activities, such as work or driving, and make preparations accordingly. Depending on the type of surgery, you may also have questions about activities such as reading, TV viewing, or engaging in sexual activity. Form 17 can be helpful in answering these questions. It also sets a plan in motion for future follow-up with the doctor.

Questions to Ask Before Surgery

Decision to Pursue Surgery as Therapeutic Choice

What is the purpose of the surgery? _____

_____

_____

What other treatments are available? Is it worth trying non-surgical
treatments first? Why is surgery being recommended over other treatments?

_____

_____

Potential Benefits

What is the best outcome I could hope for? _____

_____

_____

What is the most probable outcome? What are the statistics on the success
and failure of this procedure? What constitutes success? _____

_____

_____

How will the surgery improve the quality of my life and daily functioning?

_____

_____

Potential Risks

What is the chance of dying from this operation? _____

_____

What complications could result? How likely are they to occur? _____

_____

_____

Do I have any medical conditions that increase the risk of complications?

_____

Are repeat surgeries likely to be needed? _____

_____

Decision to Use a Specific Surgeon

What is the surgeon's level of experience with my particular condition and how many times has he performed the procedure and over what period of time? _____

_____

_____

Has the surgeon completed the medical board examinations? Is he a Fellow in the American College of Surgeons? _____

Has the doctor received any additional medical specialty board certification that recognizes additional training and experience? _____

_____

_____

What is the surgeon's success rate? _____

_____

What is the surgeon's complication rate? _____

_____

Where will the surgery be performed, and what time should I arrive at the hospital or clinic? _____

_____

Should I ask for a second opinion, and what are the names of other surgeons who could provide a second opinion? _____

_____

Before the Surgery

What preparations are needed before the surgery? _____

_____

What should I bring with me? _____

_____

_____

What should I wear? _____

If Female: Can I wear make-up and nail polish or use hair products? _____

_____

What tests will I need before the surgery—for example, blood tests, electrocardiogram? _____

_____

_____

What restrictions on medications or food are needed before entering the hospital? _____

_____

How long should I refrain from eating or drinking before surgery? _____

_____

Should I take my usual medications before surgery? _____

Can I take my usual herbal and nonprescription medications before surgery?

_____

What should I do if I do not feel well—for example, I have a cold on the day of the surgery? _____

_____

Does having my period interfere with having surgery? _____

Specifics of the Surgery

Is the surgery an outpatient or inpatient procedure? _____

What does the operation entail? Are there different ways of performing the surgery and if so, what are the risks and benefits of each approach? Why is one approach being selected over another? _____

_____

_____

Exactly who will perform the surgery? _____

_____

Blood Transfusions

Will blood transfusions be used? If so, what are the risks? Are there any alternatives—for example, donating one's own blood ahead of time or family member blood donation? _____

_____

Recovery from Surgery

Describe the recovery period. How long is the typical hospital stay? _____

_____

_____

Can I drive home? _____

Will it be necessary for a family member, friend, home health aide, or nurse to come to my home and assist me after the surgery? _____

_____

Will I need any specific equipment in my house during the recovery period?

_____

How painful is the recovery period? What will be done to control the pain?

_____

_____

_____

When can I resume eating and will there be any special diet recommendations? _____

_____

Will I be able to return to my regular activities and when? _____

_____

What follow-up will be needed after the surgery? _____

_____

Anesthesia

What kind of anesthesia will be used? What are the options? _____

_____

_____

Who will be my anesthesiologist? When do I meet the anesthesiologist?

_____

CHAPTER 23

Don't Compliment a Doctor Who Will Not Discuss Complementary Medicine

Mrs. Dobbins was seeing her internist Dr. Phillips for high blood pressure. On a recent office visit, she revealed that she was feeling depressed. Dr. Phillips prescribed the antidepressant sertraline (Zoloft®). One week later, Mrs. Dobbins was evaluated in the emergency room for confusion, jerky movements of her limbs, a racing heart beat, and severe sweating. The emergency room physician suspected the diagnosis "serotonin syndrome," a medication-induced condition due to an excess of the brain chemical serotonin.

He was at a loss however, to explain how this developed in response to low dose sertraline, until he uncovered the fact that Mrs. Dobbins had also been taking an herbal remedy, St. John's Wort. While Dr. Phillips was usually very thorough about reviewing his patients' list of medications, he was not accustomed to inquiring about alternative medicines. Mrs. Dobbins was also disinclined to mention her herbal therapies, concluding that a traditional doctor would not be very interested. Unfortunately, a severe drug interaction between St. John's Wort and this antidepressant, which notoriously results in the serotonin-syndrome, could have been avoided if doctor and patient had communicated more openly.

Do you take echinacea to treat the common cold? Do you pop garlic pills? Do you undergo reflexology treatments? Have you mentioned these practices to your doctor? Alternative medicine encompasses therapies outside the standard treatment approaches used by medical doctors. Complementary medicine, such as acupuncture or chiropractic manipulations, is used to supplement rather than replace conventional treatments, but they are rarely discussed during the typical doctor-patient encounter. However, millions of Americans increasingly use some form of alternative medicine treatment. Whether the doctor accepts or rejects these therapies, the health care provider needs to know if they are being used because they may affect your health and the outcome of the treatments the doctor has prescribed.

Medical doctors are accustomed to demanding evidence of effectiveness and the safety of a medical treatment. The best form of evidence comes in the form of double-blind randomized trials in which half a group of people are assigned to receive the active treatment and half receive an inactive sugar pill; both patient and doctor are unaware of who is receiving which treatment so there is minimized bias in the interpretation of results. However, although many widely accepted traditional therapies have not been subject to these standards, an increasing amount of impressive evidence has been accumulated for alternative medicine therapies, such as ginkgo biloba for improvement of thinking function and blood flow throughout the body.

Many doctors accommodate the desire of people to use alternative medicine, so long as there are no significant drug interactions or side effects. Because doctors are often unfamiliar with these remedies, both patient and doctor should strive to obtain as much information about them as possible. *The Essentials of Complementary and Alternative Medicine* by Wayne B. Jonas and Jeffrey S. Levin is useful in this regard.

Examples of popular herbal products and their uses, and concerns doctors may have about them are listed in Table 23-1.

TABLE 23-1

Some Popular Herbal Products [13]

Method of Miriam M. Chan, R.PH., PHARM.D., *Riverside Family Practice Residency Program,* Columbus, Ohio.

Herb	Common Uses	Precautions and Drug Interactions
Black Cohosh	Commonly used to relieve menopausal symptoms, such as hot flashes. Also used to treat premenstrual discomfort and dysmenorrhea.	Black cohosh has an estrogen-like action and has been shown to decrease luteinizing hormone. Large doses of the plant may induce miscarriage; contraindicated during pregnancy. May cause gastrointestinal disturbances, headache, and hypotension. Long-term studies have not been conducted on the herb. Therefore, use should be limited to 6 months.

---

13. Excerpted from *Some Popular Herbal Products* by Miriam M.Chan, R.PH., Ph.D., pg. 1244-1245. *Conn's Current Therapy.* Edited by Robert E. Rakel, and Edward T. Bope, M.D. W.B. Saunders Company, New York, 2002.

Chamomile	Used orally to calm nerves and treat gastrointestinal spasms and inflammatory disease of the gastrointestinal tract. Used topically to treat wounds, skin infections, and skin/mucous membrane inflammations.	Chamomile may cause an allergic reaction, especially in people with severe allergies to ragweed or other members of the daisy family — for example, echinacea, feverfew, and milk thistle. It should not be taken concurrently with other sedatives, such as alcohol or benzodiazepines.
Echinacea	Used as an immune stimulant, particularly for the prevention and treatment of colds and influenza. Supportive therapy for lower urinary tract infections. Used topically to treat skin disorders and promote wound healing.	Echinacea should not be used by people with autoimmune disease. Long-term use (over 8 weeks) may suppress immunity and therefore is not recommended. Allergic reaction to echinacea has been reported. Adverse events are rare and may include mild gastrointestinal effects.
Ephedra (Ma Huang)	For diseases of the respiratory tract with mild bronchospasms Commonly found in weight-loss products. Also marketed as a stimulant for performance enhancement.	Ephedra contains ephedrine, which has sympathomimetic activities. Consequently, it should not be used by people who have cardiovascular disease, diabetes, glaucoma, hypertension, hyperthyroidism, prostate enlargement, psychiatric disorders, or seizure. Serious adverse effects, including seizures, arrhythmias, heart attack, stroke, and death, have been associated with the use of ephedra. Concurrent use of ephedra and digitalis, guanethidine, MAOs, or other stimulants, including caffeine, is not recommended.
Feverfew	For migraine headache prophylaxis. For treatment of fever, menstrual problems, and arthritis.	Feverfew may induce menstrual bleeding and is contraindicated in pregnancy. Fresh leaves may cause oral ulcers and gastrointestinal irritation. Sudden discontinuation of feverfew can precipitate rebound headache.

		Feverfew may interact with anticoagulants and potentiate the antiplatelet effect of aspirin.
Garlic	To lower blood pressure and serum cholesterol. To prevent atherosclerosis.	The intake of large quantities can lead to stomach complaints. Garlic has antiplatelet effects and may interact with anticoagulants.
Ginger	As an antiemetic. For prevention of motion sickness.	Ginger should not be used by people with gallstones because of its cholagogic effect. It may inhibit platelet aggregation. Cases of postoperative bleeding have been reported. Large doses of ginger may increase bleeding time in people who are taking antiplatelet agents.
Ginkgo Biloba	For dementia, to slow cognitive deterioration. For claudication to increase peripheral blood flow.	Adverse effects are rare and may include mild stomach or intestinal upsets, headache, or allergic skin reaction. Ginkgo can inhibit platelet aggregation. Reports of spontaneous bleeding have been published. Concurrent use of ginkgo and anticoagulants, antiplatelet agents, vitamin E, or garlic may increase risk of bleeding.
Ginseng	As a tonic in time of stress, fatigue, and debility, and during convalescence. To improve physical performance and stamina.	Ginseng has a mild stimulant effect and should be avoided by people with cardiovascular disease. Tachycardia and hypertension can occur. Overdosage can lead to *ginseng abuse syndrome*, characterized by insomnia, hypotonia, and edema. Ginseng has estrogenic effects and may cause vaginal bleeding and breast tenderness. Ginseng should not be used with other stimulants. People taking antidiabetic agents and ginseng should be monitored to avoid hypoglycemic effects of ginseng. Ginseng may interact with warfarin, causing decreased INR.

		Siberian ginseng may increase digoxin levels. There have been reports of drug interaction between ginseng and phenelzine (an MAOI) resulting in insomnia, headache, tremulousness, and manic-like symptoms.
Kava-kava	Anxiolytic for nervous anxiety, stress, and restlessness. Sedative used to induce sleep.	Contraindications include people with depression, pregnancy, and nursing mothers. Kava may affect motor reflexes and judgment when driving and/or operating heavy machinery. Accommodative disturbances have been reported. Kava may cause exacerbation of Parkinson's disease. Extended use can cause a temporary yellow discoloration of skin, hair, and nails. Kava has been shown to have additive CNS effects with other CNS depressants — for example, benzodiazepines, alcohol, or herbal tranquilizers.
Milk Thistle	As a hepatoprotectant and antioxidant, particularly for the treatment of hepatitis, cirrhosis, and toxic liver damage. Used in Europe for the treatment of hepatotoxic mushroom poisoning from *Amanita phalloides*.	Adverse effects are rare but may include diarrhea and allergic reactions. People taking antidiabetic agents and milk thistle should be monitored to avoid hypoglycemia.
Saw Palmetto	To treat urination problem in benign prostatic hyperplasia. For irritable bladder.	Adverse effects are rare but may include headache, nausea, and upset stomach. High doses can cause diarrhea.
St. John's Wort	Effective for mild to moderate depression. May have anti-inflammatory and anti-infective activities.	St. John's Wort should not be used during pregnancy. Side effects include dry mouth, gastrointestinal upset, dizziness, fatigue, and constipation. St. John's Wort may induce photosensitivity, especially in fair-skinned individuals. Caution advised if used with other antidepressants, including SSRIs or serotonergic drugs because it may cause serotonin syndrome.

		St. John's Wort has been shown to induce the P450 isoenzymes and decrease the blood levels of many drugs, such as indinavir, cyclosporine, digoxin, theophylline, oral contraceptive pills, and warfarin.
Valerian	Mild sedative for insomnia. Minor tranquilizer for nervousness.	Valerian can cause morning drowsiness. Long-term administration may lead to paradoxic stimulation, including restlessness and palpitations. It may potentiate the sedative effect of CNS depressants—for example, benzodiazepines, alcohol, and other herbal tranquilizers.

Abbreviations: CNS central nervous system; MAOI = monoamine oxidase inhibitor; SSRIs = selective serotonin reuptake inhibitors.

This chapter was not written to support or argue against the value of alternative/complementary medicine techniques and treatments. However, most doctors are concerned about the commonly held notion that these therapies are more natural and therefore completely safe. These concerns are supported by numerous reported side effects and the worry that if these therapies are used to replace conventional medical treatments serious diseases may progress in severity, perhaps even kill people.

Because many doctors are unfamiliar with alternative/complementary medicine, it is a healthy exercise for doctor and patient to investigate what is known about the proposed alternative treatment and discuss the risks and benefits openly.

The following examples are a few of the potential side effects worth a conversation with the doctor.

- Acupuncture: Discuss the possible risk of infection transmitted by acupuncture needles and rare cases of injury to important body tissues when needles are placed in sensitive areas.

- Spinal manipulation, such as chiropractic: Discuss the risk of stroke or developing a slipped disc in the spine.

- Excessive use of vitamins, animal preparations—such as bee-sting therapy or Spanish fly—toxic metals, or unusual and possibly unbalanced diets. Investigate the wide assortment of reported complications with your doctor.

- Enzyme therapy: Skin application or internal intake of substances that chemically break down other substances in the body. Discuss the risk of allergic reactions and the risk of going into shock.

- Fasting: Believed to cleanse the body. Discuss whether current illnesses, age, or being pregnant, puts you at particularly high risk for complications.
- Rolfing: This deep massage therapy is purported to improve general and emotional health. Discuss potential pain during treatment.

CHAPTER 24

Be Prepared When You Call Your Doctor

Telephone communications between patient and doctor place the greatest stress on the doctor-patient relationship. When the patient calls with an urgent problem, the doctor may need to interrupt a busy clinic schedule to answer the call and deal with the problem. If the call is less urgent, the phone call may be returned at the end of the day, a time when the doctor has completed a possibly long and exhausting day at the hospital and office. Sometimes doctors are deluged with phone calls and the stress of dealing with calls may be evident during the phone conversation. Doctors unfortunately do not always call back promptly because they are attending to other urgent matters or because they did not receive the message. Hopefully, the failure to call back is not due to lack of concern by the doctor.

Given the difficulties inherent in telephone communication, there are many things people can do to get their needs addressed in the most efficient and optimum fashion.

Take Two Aspirins and Call My Receptionist in the Morning

In many instances, it is likely that you will not be able to speak to the doctor immediately and, therefore, a message will need to be left stating concisely what your concern is. The following recommendations apply when speaking to the doctor's receptionist

- State your name clearly and spell it if necessary.
- Write down the name of the receptionist and the date and time you called. This can be helpful should your phone calls go unanswered and you or the doctor want to trace the reason a message was not received.
- State the nature of your problem clearly. This information should be prepared before picking up the phone. One sentence of background, followed by the new issue should be stated. For example: "I am followed by Dr. Jones for arthritis and I am experiencing severe joint

swelling over the past two days;" or "I see Dr. Johnson for high blood pressure and I have developed new abdominal pain since this morning."

- Offer specific questions to be addressed to the doctor, such as: Do I need to be seen in the office immediately? Can the doctor prescribe a medicine over the phone for me? Do I need to fast before I undergo the blood test ordered by the doctor?

- Leave specific information about the name of the pharmacy, including the address and phone number, if you are calling about a prescription refill. Prepare the information before calling. List the name of the medicine, spell it, and indicate exactly how it is taken (dose of each pill, how many of each pill is taken, and at what times of the day). Also provide the total amount (in milligrams) taken each day in order to confirm that the drug information is correct. If you anticipate a difference between the dosage you are currently taking and the amount listed at the pharmacy or in the doctor's record, leave information to explain the disparity.

- Leave specific phone numbers where you can be reached and then be available for the return phone call. Doctors often resent getting a message saying they expect a call-back within a very narrow time-frame—for example, "Call back between 6 and 7 p.m. tonight." The chances of receiving a return phone call sharply diminishes if you severely limit the time you are available to receive the call-back. Leave complete information with the person designated to receive the call for you if you will not be available to receive the doctor's return phone call.

When Speaking to the Doctor on the Phone

If you reach the doctor on the first try, or when the phone call is returned, all of the recommendations above are useful. Describing the problem to the doctor should be done in an organized and concise fashion. It is helpful to write down your thoughts first and then refer to them when speaking to the doctor. Tell the doctor how long the problem or symptom has been bothering you.

The content of telephone calls should be focused on the most urgent concerns; more general discussions should be left for the next office visit. Your problem is much more likely to be addressed by the doctor if you are specific and do not ramble.

Sometimes, particularly if the call is urgent and your doctor is unavailable, a nurse or another doctor may call you back. If a health care provider who is unfamiliar with your history is covering for your doctor, it is useful to mention the highlights of your medical background and then go on to describe the immediate problem. Be prepared to provide a list of medications you are taking. For example "I have seen Dr. Smith for three years for the problems of low back pain, angina, and diabetes mellitus. I have developed new dizziness today. My daily medications are Insulin, Motrin, and when needed, nitroglycerin under the tongue.

When the Doctor Does Not Call Back

There are many possible reasons for a doctor to fail to call back a patient. For routine matters, 24 to 48 hours is a reasonable waiting time. For urgent issues, a call-back may be indicated immediately. Waste no time in going to an emergency room if your problem is truly urgent. Tell the doctor your concerns about any unanswered phone calls when you finally reach him. If the doctor did not receive the message, provide her with the time, date, and person you spoke to when you left the message. Unanswered phone calls can seriously undermine a positive doctor-patient relationship, and you may want to consider consulting another doctor if your doctor repeatedly does not return your phone calls.

PART IV
Other Useful Information

Do Not Go Out of Your Mind When You Go Out of Network– Understanding Medical Insurance Plans

"I divided the medical bills into two piles – those that the insurance company paid correctly and those they had not. The ones they paid I filed away; the other ones I stuffed into my briefcase to bring to work. My employer was owned by my insurance carrier; any payment problems were work-related and would be dealt with on company time using company phones.

'What did they pay wrong?' my wife asked.

'Oh, all sorts of things,' I replied. 'They did not pay the non-network doctor everything. Something about reasonable and customary.'

'They do that so you do not go to some overpriced Hollywood doctor,' she explained.

'Yes, but they were the ones who chose that doctor.' I leafed through the pile. 'They did not pay the blood tests because they went to an out-of-network lab.'

'But those tests were done at the doctor's office,' she said. 'They have a machine right there.'

'Apparently your doctor is in the network but his equipment is not.'"

DAVID TILLMAN
In The Failing Light: A Memoir

Preparing information about your medical condition is very important, but preparing information that the doctor's office needs for billing your office visit to the insurance company is essential in order to guarantee that you will even be seen by the doctor! With the ever-confusing array of insurance plans, coming to the office equipped with the necessary information can save a lot of time and aggravation.

Let's start with the typical information you will need in hand in order to complete patient registration forms at the doctor's office.

- Your social security number and that of the insured (if the policy is under someone else's name, such as a spouse)

- Your date of birth

- Your home address and telephone number
- Your employer's name, address, and telephone number
- Your spouse and/or legal guardian's name, address, telephone number, and social security number
- The address and telephone number of the primary care doctor and the referring doctor (may be the same)
- The name, address, and telephone number of the primary and secondary insurance. (Carry your insurance cards with you at all times. You may need them in case there is an unexpected emergency.)
- The address and telephone number of each insurance company

Also, remember to bring your insurance card. It will have numbers on it that are typically requested by the doctor's office, including insurance group number, certificate number, and plan number.

Some insurance companies require that you obtain a completed referral form from your primary care doctor in order to see a specialist. It is important to make sure that the specialist is a participating doctor in your insurance plan. If not, you will typically need to ask the insurance company to authorize an *out-of-network* referral form allowing you to seek care from a nonparticipating doctor. Since seeing a health care provider without this referral sheet may result in nonpayment to the doctor, many doctors may decline to perform a service without it. The authorization will identify the type, number, and duration of services covered for that episode of care. Patients should discuss their authorization status with the doctor's office on a regular basis in order to ensure that future services are covered.

There are a wide variety of medical insurance plans, each with its own advantages and disadvantages. In the following section, we summarize issues raised in an excellent review found in *Health Insurance Resources: A Guide for People with a Chronic Disease or Disability.*

Indemnity insurance, also referred to as fee-for-service coverage—refers to the traditional form of insurance that was prevalent before managed care became dominant. People with fee-for-service insurance may be responsible for paying the percentage of the doctor's fee that is not covered by the insurance plan. The advantage of indemnity insurance is the relative lack of limitation on the doctors or hospitals covered by the plan. You can be evaluated at virtually any doctor's office or hospital in the country, and you can change health care providers anytime. These plans have variability in their coverage of prescription drugs and out-of-hospital care. Many people have moved away from this type of insurance, however, because the cost for this insurance is substantially higher than managed care plans and some services may not be as well covered. People with indemnity insurance should check to what extent the doctor's visit or procedures ordered by the doctor are covered by their plan. Such insurance plans typically have a *deductible*, a set amount of money per year that is spent on tests, doctor visits, or procedures, before the insurance company coverage kicks in. Deductibles are typically in the range of $500 or less.

Managed care refers to an organizational approach that coordinates both the provisional care and its financing. One of its goals is to produce high quality care, while reducing the costs associated with it. This can be achieved through the use of negotiated rates (pre-paid capitated arrangements with providers), health care resource utilization, and participation in quality improvement programs. The classic model of managed care is the Health Maintenance Organization (HMO). With this type of insurance plan, you see a doctor who is directly employed and paid by the HMO, an independent doctor who has a contract with the HMO, or a doctor belonging to a multispecialty group that has contracted with the HMO. A variation of this is belonging to a *preferred provider organization* (PPO) in which doctors agree to provide services at reduced rates but are still paid on a fee-for-service basis. If a person wants to see a non-preferred, out-of-network doctor, they usually have to pay a higher rate when using those particular doctors. People do not have to choose how to receive services, or from whom, until the need arises in *point of service* plans.

The advantages of managed care plans include reduced costs to gain coverage, and the care provided by HMOs is comprehensive, including doctor's visits, hospitalizations, emergency care, surgery, and other treatments. Employers may cover the costs for enrolling in managed care programs. Claim forms do not need to be submitted to the insurance company when enrolled in a PPO, HMO, or Point of Service plan by the person who received the services. The disadvantages include more limitations and less flexibility in the choice of health care providers and in the tests and procedures that are ordered.

In managed care plans, the insured typically chooses a primary care provider who serves as a gatekeeper for approving or disapproving evaluation by and recommendations of a specialist. Typically, a doctor who wants to perform a procedure, surgery, or test needs authorization from the health plan. Some health plans require that tests or services be performed at contracted facilities, and failure to adhere to these guidelines may result in nonpayment of services. Even off-label uses of a drug may not be covered. (*Off-label* means the use of a medication for purposes beyond what the FDA has approved it for. Off-label uses are very common, because the pre-marketing testing may have been just sufficient enough to get it marketed, whereas, post-marketing experience demonstrated the drug's effectiveness in many other conditions.)

Form 18 provides a list of questions that are useful to ask when selecting an insurance program. Make multiple copies of this form and ask each insurance company representative these questions when deciding on a plan, write in the answers, and compare them.

Medicare and Medicaid

Medicare is the federal health insurance program for people over the age of 65 and for certain people with disabilities. Medicare Part A covers hospitalizations, durable medical equipment, and certain supplies; Part B covers doctor visits, procedures, and some supplies ordered by the doctor. Medicare does not cover prescription drugs and has specific requirements with regards to long-term care, such as skilled nursing home care. Medicare reimburses doctors for services on a fee-for-service basis. Reimbursement is dependent on the complexity, duration, and type of service performed by the doctor.

Medicaid is another federally-supported health care coverage that is provided only to individuals with limited financial resources and income. In contrast to Medicare, Medicaid does cover the cost of prescriptions, but many doctors do not accept Medicaid because the reimbursements to doctors are very low.

Work with your Doctor to Get Insurance Approval for Tests, Procedures, and Treatment

With the current focus on reducing health-care costs, many insurers place restrictions and close scrutiny on expensive tests and procedures. Frustrations abound concerning difficulties getting some tests or treatments covered. Several important guidelines should be followed in seeking test or treatment coverage:

1. The primary care doctor usually needs to approve a test, procedure, or treatment. If he does not approve the recommended test or procedure, have the doctor requesting the services provide detailed information to the primary care doctor and, ideally, have them speak personally so the need for approval is understood. Sometimes, the requesting doctor may need to call the insurance company directly. Insurance companies typically use the concept of *medical necessity* as the criterion for approval and, therefore, good documentation supporting the medical necessity for a test or procedure should be provided. Be prepared to furnish the specialist with all of the necessary contact information, including the name, telephone number, and address of the specific contact person at the insurance company or the contact information necessary to reach your primary care doctor.

2. Calling insurance companies can be a frustrating experience. If you call the company yourself and you are not satisfied with the person you speak with, ask to speak to the supervisor. Do not take no for an answer.

3. Consult written materials provided by the insurance company for appealing any denials of tests or procedures.

4. If appealing to the insurance company is unsuccessful, contact your employer to inform them of your dissatisfaction with the company. Also notify the appropriate state agencies, including your state's Department of Insurance or State Insurance Appeals Board. In certain circumstances, you may consider contacting a consumer advocate, such as someone in the media, or your local congressman.

FORM 18

Questions to Ask
Before You Enroll in a Managed Care Plan

What does the plan cover? _____

_____

_____

Does the plan cover adjunct services, such as dental, optometry, mental health counseling, prescription medication, and substance abuse treatment programs? _____

_____

What will my monthly premium be, and what portion will my employer pay, if any? _____

Is there a deductible or co-payment for services? What is the maximum out-of-pocket? Are there annual or lifetime maximums on deductibles? ____

_____

Is there a limit to the number of visits for specific services that will be covered—for example, mental health, home health care, or transplantation?

_____

_____

Does the plan exclude any preexisting conditions? Which ones and for how long? _____

Can I choose my primary care doctor? If I am not satisfied, will I be able to switch doctors? _____

How many of the doctors in the plan are board-certified? _____

_____

If I already have a doctor, is she one of the participating providers in the plan? _____

Is the primary care doctor's office convenient to my home or office, and are the hours convenient for me and my family? _____

How long will the typical waiting time be for a new appointment with my primary care doctor? _____

Does the plan allow me to access doctors outside the network? Will I have to pay extra if I use doctors outside the plan? _____

Are the hospitals I might use part of the managed care plan's network? ____

_____

What are the procedures for reimbursement for emergency care? _____

_____

Does the plan have a grievance procedure to challenge claims that are not allowed? _____

Is the plan certified by the NCQA (National Committee for Quality Assurance)? _____

How long will it take to get an appointment with a primary care doctor? ___

_____

Where would I be referred for specialty care? _____

How much of the plan's budget is spent on administrative costs and profit, and how much for patient care? _____

CHAPTER 26

You Do Not Have to Be a Doctor to Get a Medical Education – Ignorance is Not Bliss When It Comes to Your Health

"Over a two-year period I saw seven different doctors in search of a diagnosis for my symptoms. I fell through the cracks every step of the way. It did not matter that I was the Nanny and everyone loved the show. I did not know what to ask for, and I was not offered all available tests that could have diagnosed me. So for two years I walked around with a progressively worsening cancer and none of these doctors, not one, offered me the simple test that ultimately detected it. Maybe they thought I was too young. Too young for uterine cancer, but just ripe for a perimenopausal hormone imbalance. Please, I could not accept I was beginning my menopause at the very moment I was single and entering my sexual peak! No way. And thank God I did not, because nothing could have been further from the truth.

We need to educate ourselves about our bodies. Women need to understand gynecological cancers and the tests that can help detect them. We should know what's out there. We should hear our options. We should be in control. Once you wake up and smell the coffee, it is hard to go back to sleep! Let me sound the alarm. Since it is not my intention to point fingers at individual doctors, I do not name the names of those doctors I went to along the way. They're no different, no better, no worse, than the doctors you may encounter in your neck of the woods. It is not about them, it is about you. *US*. We're the ones who must change, if we ever expect there to be change. We have to take control of the situation, become educated consumers, network among ourselves, and gain information and insight into getting diagnosed and getting treatment. Someone gimme a podium!"

FRAN DRESCHER
Cancer Schmancer

"After I arrive at a diagnosis, the next step is to allow the patient to become a partner in deciding how to confirm the diagnosis and what course of treatment to follow. One of my primary roles as an internist is to educate patients about their illness. I typically discuss preventive measures, the origins of the disease, and both the benefits and possible side effects of the medication they may use. In doing this, I ask that the patients become more responsible for their health. When patients are well informed, they are more compliant and interested in maintaining their health."

ERIN CARDON
From The Mind/Body Connection in My First Year As a Doctor: Real-World Stories From America's M.D.s

The primary purpose of this book is to help you prepare personal information and questions for your doctor, but another very important way to prepare for the doctor's visit is to enhance your knowledge about symptoms, diagnoses, tests, and treatments. Currently, there are numerous avenues for gaining medical information; some are excellent, and others are fraught with danger. In *Making Informed Medical Decisions: Where to Look and How to Use What You Find* by N. Oster, L. Thomas, and D. Joseff, the authors enumerate resources for obtaining medical information. In the following discussion, we highlight some of the points they raise, as well as our own opinions about these sources of information.

Academic Medical Libraries

Academic medical libraries based at universities and medical centers typically have an abundance of written materials on medical subjects. However, most of the available texts and articles are written for trained health care providers and use medical jargon that may be difficult for the layperson to understand. This could lead to further unnecessary anxiety about medical conditions. Medical textbooks tend to be conservative in their recommendations and are sometimes slightly outdated, given the amount of time it takes for publications to receive contributions by various authors and reach hardcopy publication. In general, medical textbooks offer excellent general reviews on a topic.

In contrast, journals tend to be more up-to-date, and most journal articles undergo a process called *peer-review*, in which experts in a given area are asked to anonymously comment and rate scientific submissions to a journal. However, some journals have much less rigorous criteria, particularly if the journal does not have sufficient articles to fill a given issue. Among treatment studies, the most convincing evidence comes from studies utilizing what are called *placebo-controlled, double-blind trials*, in which people randomly receive either an active treatment or a sugar-pill, and neither the patient nor the doctor are aware what is being given to a specific person. This reduces the bias associated with hopeful expectations about a treatment. Conversely, the weakest evidence comes from single case reports.

Newspapers may publish highlights of studies and disease updates even before the medical journal article goes to print.

Hospital Libraries

Hospital libraries, similar to academic medical libraries, are also based at a medical center or teaching hospital. Many hospital libraries have extended their collections to include patient education resources, such as books and online health databases. Many hospital libraries encourage public use of the library's consumer health resources, and some even have consumer health specialists in addition to the staff librarian.

Public Libraries

Public libraries have texts and magazines that are directed more toward the layperson, and the accuracy of the information conveyed varies widely. Many books are disease-specific; others provide comprehensive guides to general medical diagnosis and treatment. We prefer a number of the medical school-based medical health guides, such as the *Harvard Medical School Family Health Guide* or the *Johns Hopkins Family Health Book.*

Consumer health magazines are very useful for translating complex medical knowledge into an easily understood format, but accuracy and reliability of the information is not always the best. Other written information, including newsletters, such as *The Harvard Health Letter*, health pamphlets, and reports from the media may be available at public libraries as well from many of the sources listed below.

Public libraries also have computerized databases devoted to consumer health information. *The Health Reference Center* is a well-known database that permits access to references on a wide assortment of health topics. Free access to consumer health information is available via the Internet on Medlineplus (the layperson's version of Medline used by doctors) at www.medlineplus.gov or New York Online Access to Health at www.noah-health.org. Some major public libraries have separate consumer health information centers that are supervised by medical librarians or consumer health specialists.

Bookstores

Local bookstores have texts and magazines for the layperson that are similar to those found at public libraries. University and medical school bookstores are more likely to carry medical textbooks. Internet bookstores tend to carry books written for health care providers and the lay public.

Government Agencies

Government agencies, such as the National Institute of Health, offer abundant public information on a wide range of medical issues. Such organizations can be contacted by phone, by mail, and via the Internet.

Professional Associations

Professional associations include medical organizations catering to health care providers who are focused on different disorders or disciplines of medicine. Some of these organizations have websites that include a diversity of information that can be accessed. Some organizations divide their resources into those for health care providers and those for the lay public.

Nonprofit organizations are often disease-specific agencies, usually directed toward the lay public. They are interested in promoting knowledge and advancements in the treatment of a specific disorder. Many of these agencies are eager to provide information via mailings, telephone contacts, and the Internet. Some of the information conveyed may be based on individual experience rather than rigorously scientifically tested recommendations. These agencies can be located on the Internet, through directories of health care organizations, and through local health departments.

Patient Resource Centers

These centers are often disease-specific and are found at different locations throughout the country. They are independent or sometimes affiliated with a medical center. These centers often feature collections of books, videotapes, and an assortment of written materials. They may also be able to put you in contact with other people who have the same medical condition as you, and who are willing to share their knowledge and experience.

Medical Research Centers

Science and clinical researchers who are focused on a given disease are often experts on that particular disorder and may be conducting relevant investigations. These experts may be identified by their presence in the medical literature, including being invited to write chapters in leading medical textbooks.

Medical Product Manufacturers

Companies that produce treatment options often amass information about the conditions treated by their products. This information may be very informative, although it should be interpreted cautiously because there may be an underlying bias toward emphasizing the value of the given product for the specific disease. Each pharmaceutical company has a "1-800-..." telephone number for consumers that can usually be found in the *Physician's Desk Reference* (PDR) or on the Internet.

Internet

The Internet is an extraordinary source of medical health information and excels in providing information about breaking medical news, recent journal articles, drug information, and tidbits of medical knowledge from many different sources. Web chat rooms provide an opportunity for individuals to communicate anonymously with others who are experiencing similar problems in order to share knowledge and advice. Medical journal search engines are also increasingly available through the Internet. Unfortunately, information from the Internet is best likened to blaring music instruments in an orchestra without a conductor. While some information sources attempt to select the most evidence-based data, other sources publish mostly untested opinions or advertisements disguised as scientific information. Some older websites may convey information that is no longer accurate. Caution is therefore advised when reviewing Internet-based medical knowledge.

Listed below are some of the websites that offer general health information:

http://webmd.com

http://www.thirdage.com/health/

http://healthlinkplus.org/

http://medlineplus.adam.com/

http://chid.nih.gov/

http://caphis.mlanet.org/consumer/index.html

http://www.emedicine.com/

http://healthanswers.com/

http://www.healthatoz.com/

http://www.intelihealth.com/IH/ihtIH

http://www.mayoclinic.com/index.cfm

http://medhlp.netusa.net/search.htm

http://www.merckhomeedition.com/home.html

http://locatorplus.gov/

http://consumer.pdr.net/index.html

http://personalmd.com/

http://healthnewsdirectory.com

http://www.nlm.nih.gov/medlineplus/tutorials.html

http://yoursurgery.com/index.cfm

http://rxlist.com/

http://www.health.harvard.edu/fhg/diagnostics.shtml

Doctors: The Good, the Bad, and the Ugly–Do Not Let Difficult Doctors Get On Your Case[14]

> "If I had to guess, I would say that the principal contribution made by my doctor to the taming, and possibly the conquest, of my illness was that he encouraged me to believe I was a respected partner with him in the total undertaking. He fully engaged my subjective energies. He may not have been able to define or diagnose the process through which self-confidence (wild hunches securely believed) was somehow picked up by the body's immunologic mechanisms and translated into antimorbid effects, but he was acting, I believe, in the best tradition of medicine in recognizing that he had to reach out in my case beyond the usual verifiable modalities. In so doing, he was faithful to the first dictum in his medical education: above all, do not harm."
>
> NORMAN COUSINS
> *Anatomy of an Illness as Perceived by the Patient:*
> *Reflections on Healing and Regeneration*

It is difficult to find a good doctor, one who offers a combination of compassion, caring, sensitivity, dedication, intelligence, and competence. Some people say that it is easier to shop for a car than it is to find the best doctor. After all, you could investigate the qualities of the car by reviewing numerous consumer guides, meet with a sales representative, and even give it a test drive. Giving a doctor a test drive is a little more challenging. Form 19 can be used to help you focus on what you need in a physician. Make multiple copies for comparison if you are considering more than one.

Difficult Doctors

> "Saint Peter is showing a visitor around heaven. While he is explaining to him that, contrary to popular belief, God's function is only that of chairman of the board and that he has no influence on anything that happens in the universe, they come upon him sitting in front of a giant microscope. As he barks orders, such as 'So-and-so has to die,'

14. Adapted in part from: (1) *Doctor-Patient Interactions. In: Smart Patient Good Medicine* by R.L. Sribnick and W.B. Sribnick. New York: Walker and Company, 1994:108-121; and (2) *Communication. In: Working with your Doctor* by N. Keene. Cambridge: O'Reilly, 1998:75-102.

'XYZ has to be pulled out at the last second,' and 'The flu epidemic is to stop today,' the visitor turns to his guide and says, 'I thought you told me that God does not have any direct executive power!' Saint Peter answers, with a finger to his lips, 'Shh, not so loud! Today's *his* day to play doctor.'"

P.H. BERCZELLER
Doctors and Patients: What We Feel About You

Just as the American Hospital Association has established *A Patient's Bill of Rights*, which is posted in hospitals across the country for inpatients and their families, we believe many of the elements contained therein should also be respected in the outpatient setting. Anyone who seeks medical attention is entitled to:

- Considerate and respectful care
- Current and understandable information concerning diagnosis, treatment, and prognosis
- The right to make decisions about plan of care
- Confidentiality

Ironically, the medical literature is filled with articles and even books about how to handle *difficult patients*—usually angry, demanding patients who are considered a nightmare to deal with. However, what about *difficult doctors*, who do not necessarily promote these fundamental rights of patients? In fact, it is very hard to find articles about "difficult doctors" in the journals and textbooks that doctors read. Yet, we have all had difficulties with doctors in one way or another. Let's turn the tables to better understand the styles of difficult doctors and ways to deal with them. Although the following categories are not an established classification of doctor types, the authors' anecdotal experience and that of their colleagues generated this information:

"Doctor God"

You may be comforted and feel you are in good hands when your doctor is self-assured and confident. However, sometimes these virtues are taken to the extreme. This type of doctor considers it beneath his dignity to get medical advice from others and almost never recommends getting a second opinion. You end up feeling as if your observations and opinions have no value. You are often too inhibited to ask the doctor very many questions. When you do question the doctor's strategy or request a second opinion, this type of doctor gets irritated. If you do get another opinion, this type of doctor avoids spending "precious time" conferring with the second doctor. It is ironic that some of the best experts in medicine recognize their limitations and understand the value of dialogue with other doctors, but Doctor God will not talk to anyone who might question his authority.

Another type of Doctor God is the one who attempts to treat everything without proper consultation. For example, this doctor will dispense numerous antidepressants to treat depression but does not refer the patient or a psychiatrist, or even simply confer with a psychiatrist.

Suggestions

Ask your doctor the relevant questions suggested in this book and insist on the getting the answers you need in order to make informed decisions. Specific suggestions about asking for a second opinion are highlighted in Chapter 20. You may want to consider switching to a more accommodating health care provider if your doctor is hostile to the idea of answering questions.

The "Nervous About Lawsuits" Doctor

Medical lawsuits abound and doctors are understandably concerned about the risk of being sued for malpractice. However, some doctors are so obsessed with medical-legal risks that it leads to rampant ordering of tests in order to document that every diagnostic possibility was covered, no matter how irrelevant. They may think they have covered their "you-know-whats," but they actually often get into more trouble when excessive testing picks up incidental findings that must be explained as well.

Suggestions

Refer to the questions in Chapter 12 about the purpose of tests, and insist that your doctor tell you how the test results will alter diagnosis and future treatments.

The "Rushed" Doctor

This doctor conveys his desire to rush through the office visit by her body language, by severely limiting comments, or by frequently interrupting you. Sometimes, this type of doctor skimps on taking a thorough history or performing a complete examination, or leaves the entire evaluation in the hands of an assistant.

Suggestions

You may need to tell this type of doctor that you feel frustrated because you do not have enough time to discuss the issues that are important to you. You may want to negotiate a more optimal appointment time when your doctor is less pressed and can give you more of his time and attention. However, this may be the fundamentally inherent style of your doctor, and if it prevents you from getting the attention that you feel is needed, you may need to look for another doctor.

The "Hostile or Argumentative" Doctor

Hopefully, this type of doctor is rare, and if you have encountered such a doctor, we are very sorry to hear it. This type of doctor displays little professionalism in dealing with the occasional conflicts that occur between patient and doctor. Instead of handling disagreements in a neutral and composed fashion, this doctor becomes nasty and may even yell at a patient. (See Chapter 28 for information about the feelings you may experience when you meet with a hostile or argumentative doctor.)

Suggestions

It is imperative to keep your cool and handle yourself in a neutral, controlled fashion, even if the doctor is unprofessional. We recommend that you attempt to calmly explain your point of view, and if the difficulty cannot be settled, move on to another doctor.

The "Detached" Doctor

This type of doctor appears to be indifferent to the emotional component of your symptoms or the anxieties that you experience. This doctor may answer all your questions, but rarely offers information spontaneously and appears to have little true interest in your symptoms. Sometimes, this is an episodic phenomenon relating to lingering distractions thinking about other cases, mental or physical exhaustion, or sometimes even depression. Alternatively, some doctors unfortunately simply do not have caring attitudes.

Suggestion

It is impossible to change a doctor's fundamental personality, and your decision to stay with a doctor should be dependent in part on whether your overall needs are being addressed to your satisfaction.

The "Anxious" Doctor

This type of doctor tries very hard but somehow ends up inspiring little confidence. It is great that she spends so much time talking with her patients. However, you might realize that she is looking to you to relieve her anxieties and uncertainties about what to do next. Some of these doctors order dozens of tests without a coherent strategy.

Suggestions

Doctors are often under immense pressures related to their clinical work and sometimes overwhelming concerns about avoiding crucial mistakes. Use the information in this book to help you decide when a second opinion is needed to supplement your doctor's recommendations and ask the appropriate questions to better understand the value of the tests that are ordered.

The "Never Call-Back" Doctor

These doctors may be very good in the office, even spending extraordinary amounts of time answering questions and explaining things. However, because of disorganization, being overextended, or frank disregard for the importance of communication with the patient, these doctors are unreliable about returning telephone calls or completing other tasks, such as writing up forms you need.

Suggestions

See Chapter 24 for more information about calling your doctor. When you meet in the office, alert your doctor to any difficulties you have experienced in getting him to return your telephone calls and try to reach a mutually agreeable strategy for dealing with future calls.

The "Don't Worry; It's Nothing" Doctor

When you are anxious about a symptom or test result and you ask your doctor about it, a reply such as "Don't worry about it" is not comforting. Most of us would feel a lot better if we understood why our difficulties are nothing to worry about and what the symptom or test really means. This phrase is often used by doctors who are in a hurry or who have a condescending attitude toward the capacity of their patients to be active partners in their medical care. This phrase may also be heard from Doctor God, described earlier. Variants of this phrase are "Oh, it's just aging," or "He'll grow out of it with time."

Suggestions

Tell your doctor that you appreciate his attempts to reassure you, but indicate that you would feel a lot better if you understood why your symptoms or test results "are nothing to worry about."

The "Limited Information" Doctor

This is sometimes a manifestation of the "detached doctor" or the "rushed doctor." This type of doctor is nice enough when questions are asked, but offers limited information spontaneously. Even essential potential risks and benefits of a treatment may be omitted unless you raise the issue.

Suggestions

The style of this type of doctor flies in the face of the spirit of this book. If your doctor does not spontaneously offer essential information, make sure you take an active stance by asking the crucial questions using the forms in this book as a guide.

The "Entrepreneurial" Doctor

This type of doctor orders numerous tests with dubious value because the doctor or the practice he belongs to owns the testing machine and can profit considerably from billing for the test procedure and its interpretation.

Suggestions

Be very wary of this when you are sent for multiple tests, one after another. In accordance with suggestions in Chapter 12, insist that your doctor explain why each test is necessary and how it will affect your diagnosis and treatment.

The "Doctor Who Speaks in Foreign Tongues"

The foreign language we are referring to is medical jargon, the terms that sound like Greek unless you have undergone formal medical training. Using medical terminology may make the doctor feel superior in stature, but it greatly impedes a healthy doctor-patient relationship and denies you the opportunity to understand your illness.

Suggestions

Insist that your doctor clarify in layman's terms what is meant by the medical terminology. Ask her to draw a diagram if appropriate and provide you with additional information that has been written for the lay public on the subject.

The "Keep You Waiting Forever in the Waiting Room" Doctor

Despite the frustration of spending extended time in the waiting room, it can be a positive sign, because it shows your doctor is devoted to spending time with each person and explaining everything in detail. Sometimes, waiting is unavoidable if an emergency call comes in or if the doctor needs to spend extra time with a prior patient in distress. It is also reasonable to be kept waiting if you have requested to be squeezed to a busy appointment schedule. However, if the wait is extreme and occurs with every office visit, it may mean your doctor is disorganized and overextended. Sometimes, these doctors arrange for unreasonable double-booking in an already busy schedule, and some of them never return telephone calls.

Suggestions

Try to determine the least busy time to have an appointment. Frequently, this is the first appointment of the day or the first visit in the afternoon following the lunch break. Always come prepared to the doctor's office with reading materials and things to do while you wait. Keep track of how many times you are kept waiting for an inordinate amount of time. We recommend you politely inform your doctor about the problem and ask if anything can be done to reduce your waiting time on subsequent appointments.

The "Constantly Interrupting" Doctor

Doctors occasionally need to interrupt patients in order to focus attention on the main points of the visit and to direct the conversation in a way that helps arrive at a diagnosis. This can be very frustrating and demeaning when the interruptions occur to an extreme degree. Doctors who frequently interrupt you may be in a hurry or may simply have their own agenda, with little regard for what you have to say.

Suggestions

Try to determine whether your doctor is reasonably redirecting the conversation in the appropriate direction or is simply rushing you for his own reasons. If it is the latter, tell the doctor that you would prefer to spend a little more time explaining what you consider to be the key issues. Keep in mind that you may not be able to discuss everything you have on your mind and may need to defer some less important issues to another visit.

The "Deficient Interviewer" Doctor

There are many types of deficiencies in the quality of medical history-taking in which the doctor fails to take a complete history. One type is taking a history comprised solely of a checklist of yes or no questions that give no room for thoughtful reflection or open-ended discussions. Another type of history-taking is dominated by leading questions in which the question makes an assumption and then asks for a yes or no response—for example, "You did not have weakness on that day, did you?" Another example is rapid-firing of questions without giving you a chance to answer each question completely. Another common problem is using expressions that make you feel as if you are being blamed for your disease—for example, saying you did not respond to the chemotherapy, rather than the cancer did not respond to the chemotherapy. Another deficiency in taking the medical history is the failure to delve into topics that are delicate or embarrassing for both doctor and patient, such as sexuality and psychosocial difficulties.

Suggestions

By using the numerous guides in this book when preparing your medical history, you may be able to combat some of these deficiencies in history-taking. Try to convey to your doctor what you consider to be the salient issues related to your medical symptoms by providing the information you have prepared in advance.

The "Psychiatrist-Bashing" Doctor

These doctors are contemptuous of psychiatry, the psychological affects of illness, or the contribution of psychological factors to medical conditions. They do a great disservice to people who are silently suffering from significant psychological distress, who will never be referred on for greatly needed psychiatric interventions. This type of doctor tends to prescribe psychiatric medications without consulting with an expert.

Suggestions

Do not wait for your doctor to recommend psychological services if you are feeling depressed or have other symptoms of psychological distress. Ask your doctor to give you a referral to a highly competent psychiatrist who is well-versed in your particular problem. If your general practitioner or nonpsychiatric specialist prescribes psychotropic medication, ask him if this treatment should be supplemented by a consultation with a psychiatrist.

The "Jokester"

This type of doctor makes you laugh by telling jokes throughout your examination and evaluation, and it can be fun. The problem occurs when the joking spirit is relentless and prevents you from sharing feelings that are not so funny, such as your fears and distress over your symptoms.

Suggestions

It is fine if you are comfortable with the lighthearted spirit of this type of doctor, but if you feel inhibited to express feelings of distress, tell your doctor that you want to discuss your more serious feelings. Try to gauge whether she changes the mood of the interview appropriately or appears to be insensitive to your request.

The "Overly Involved" Doctor

This type of doctor is sometimes beloved by his patients for trying so hard. Yet, in his zeal to provide caring service, this type of doctor fails to set realistic limits as to what can be delivered and ultimately ends up terribly overextended.

Suggestions

Try to be realistic about what your doctor can provide and what is beyond reasonable limits. Your doctor will also appreciate your consideration of his time and your attempt to work together in a friendly fashion.

The "Cocky Junior" Doctor

This type of doctor in training (intern or resident) has an arrogant attitude and does not like it when you insist on getting your information directly from the attending doctor. This type of doctor does not facilitate your discussion with the senior doctors and feels that his opinion should be enough. The Cocky Junior Doctor also does not like it when you inquire as to whether the attending doctor is performing most of your surgery or when you do not want to sign a consent form without clarifying further issues.

Suggestions

Teaching hospitals are predicated on the education of junior doctors and offer a number of advantages to patients, including an academic environment for exchange of medical information and the possibility of learning more about medical conditions by meeting a wider variety of health care providers. On the other hand, your attending doctor is ultimately in charge of your care and if there are any uncertainties in the management of your medical problems, you are entitled to communicate directly with the senior doctor.

Summary: What Can You Do?

Difficulties arising in the doctor-patient relationship need to be discussed politely, but firmly. An example, might be "Doctor, I am experiencing a little frustration trying to explain the full extent of my current problem with back pain. May I take a few uninterrupted moments to go into more detail?" You can politely ask that technical medical terms be clarified. Taking notes can be helpful, and having a friend or family member present may also be useful. Tell your doctor about any rude treatment by receptionists or other ancillary staff. Your doctor may be unaware of these problems and hopefully will make an attempt to rectify them.

Another important principle that promotes a good doctor-patient relationship is expressing appreciation for the doctor's efforts. Most doctors truly try to do their best and want their patients to feel gratified with the results of their efforts. These hard efforts occur in the face of currently great adversities in the practice of medicine, including severely reduced reimbursements from insurance companies, increased paperwork related to billing, pressures related to malpractice suits, the need to keep up with the exploding field of medicine, typically very long hours spent in the office, and many other factors. Express your appreciation to your doctor if you feel she deserves it.

Sometimes, despite the patient's and perhaps the doctor's best attempts to maintain a healthy relationship, the chemistry between patient and doctor is unhealthy. In such cases, it may be necessary to move on to another doctor.

FORM 19

Questions for Selecting a Doctor [15]

Doctor Qualifications

Did the doctor do residency training in the specific field that he currently practices in? Is the doctor board-certified; has he satisfied a list of training requirements and passed a specific examination in that field? When and where did the doctor go to medical school and train in a specific field? Was it at a university-based hospital or one with a fine reputation? _____

_____

_____

_____

Does the doctor have a medical school affiliation? Is the doctor on the teaching staff? _____

How much experience does the doctor have with my specific medical problem? _____

_____

Has the doctor been the subject of any disciplinary action? (Check your state's medical society website.) _____

_____

Referrals to a Doctor

Have any friends or family members seen the doctor? What were their impressions with regard to competence and bedside manner? Has more than one person said favorable things about the doctor? _____

_____

_____

---

15. Adapted in part from *Top Doctors: New York Metro Area.* New York: Castle Connolly Medical Ltd., 2002, and *Consumer's Guide to Top Doctors* by the editors of *Consumer's Checkbook Magazine.* 2002. Center for the Study of Services. Washington, pg. 13-14.

Does my primary doctor feel this referral is the best doctor for my condition, or was the doctor referred simply because she works at the same medical center as he does? _____

_____

Am I depending on general directories, such as hospital referral lines or advertisements, which do not necessarily screen for the best-qualified doctors? _____

Office and Hospital Issues

Is the doctor currently accepting new patients? _____

_____

How convenient is it to get to the doctor's office? Is it easily accessible by public transportation? Is it wheelchair accessible? _____

_____

Does the doctor practice solo or in a group? If the latter, will I see the same doctor each time I come, or will I be assigned to varying doctors? _____

_____

_____

What are the office hours? Does the doctor see people on weekends or evenings? _____

Will I be able to reach the doctor directly during an emergency, or will I be connected to another doctor or nondoctor? Will my doctor come to hospital if I am brought to the emergency room or hospitalized? _____

_____

How long does it usually take to get an appointment for the initial visit or for subsequent nonemergency visits? _____

Does the doctor have admitting privileges at the hospital I am most likely to be brought to in case of an emergency? _____

Insurance and Billing Issues

What is the fee for new and follow-up office visits? How much is covered by my health plan? Is the doctor connected to my health plan? _____

_____

Will the doctor take my insurance? Will the doctor accept the health plan or Medicare coverage in full? _____

_____

Will the doctor bill me or the insurance company first? _____

_____

CHAPTER 28

Feelings You May Have When You See the Doctor[16]

> "I can still see the doctor's face. He seemed delighted at his discovery when he said, 'You either have a brain tumor or Parkinson's disease. I don't think it's a brain tumor, but if it is, it's benign. I'll want you to have a CAT scan to rule it out.' His face took on a supercilious grin. 'It's such a good time to have Parkinson's disease as we have so many excellent drugs now that control it. We seldom get to see Parkinson's at such an early stage.' ... 'You know, Mrs. Grady, part of being alive is being ill, and the sooner you get used to that, the better off you'll be. I can put you on some medication called Symmetrel. It works for people with Parkinson's, but we don't know why. I think it will improve your tennis game.'
>
> I leaned across his desk, definitely in his space, about three inches from his nose, 'What we are talking about here, Dr. Anderson, is not my tennis game, but my whole fucking life.'"
>
> J. GRADY-FITCHETT
> *Flying Lessons: On The Wings of Parkinson's Disease*

When we go to the doctor, we bring not only our symptoms but also our personalities and our unique reactions to the way the doctor conducts the medical evaluation. Many people have styles of communicating their feelings that lend themselves to healthy communication with the doctor. However, other feelings may be experienced that produce obstacles in the doctor-patient relationship. Furthermore, when we are the family member accompanying our parent or spouse to the doctor, we may observe our loved ones displaying these personality styles and be concerned and troubled by them. Potential problem areas are highlighted in the following discussion as well as suggestions for how to handle them.

Anxiety

Feeling anxious is a normal emotion that is often experienced when we see the doctor. Sources of anxiety include fear of the unknown, thinking about the

16. Adapted in part from (1) *Seal up the Mouth of Outrage: Interactive Problems in Interviewing The Medical Interview: Mastering Skills for Clinical Practice* by J.L. Coulehan and M.R. Block. Philadelphia: F.A. Davis Company, 1997:183-211; and (2) *Difficult Relationships. A Guide to The Clinical Interview* by D. Levinson. Philadelphia: W.B. Saunders Company, 1987:181-196.

consequences of having a symptom or diagnosis, fear of pain, fear of being incapacitated, feeling helpless, and feeling uncertain about the future. Sometimes the anxiety relates to the reluctance to express feelings of anger about the disease or even anger toward the health care provider.

Anxiety can interfere with our ability to concentrate during office visits, impede memory, and be a major source of distraction. Completing the forms outlined in the other chapters of this book will help ensure that essential issues are addressed in spite of feeling nervous. You might experience sweating, cold hands, restlessness, flushing in the face, stuttering speech, and mild to severe degrees of trembling when you feel anxious. The astute doctor should detect these clues and adjust her interview style accordingly, including slowing down the pace of the interview, keeping a calm demeanor, showing empathy, explaining the reasons for ordering even routine tests, and inquiring about and answering patient concerns. It is appropriate to talk about your feelings and discuss the issues you are most worried about.

Anger Toward the Doctor

At one time or another, many of us experience feelings of disappointment, frustration, or outright anger toward a doctor whether we express it or not. Sometimes, feeling angry results from the perception that the primary health care provider or other staff members in a medical facility are inconsiderate, minimize our distress, or do not communicate adequately. You may feel angry that the doctor does not seem to be paying attention to the aspects of your medical condition that you believe are important and seems, instead, to emphasize other areas. It is perfectly appropriate and important to raise these issues with the doctor.

Alternatively, on other occasions, our anger toward the doctor may have more to do with our own frustration, feelings of helplessness, fears about our medical condition or even anger over circumstances not directly related to the doctor. We may even irrationally hold our health care providers to be responsible for our medical condition. Recognizing these potential sources of anger is much more difficult to do.

Caution is strongly advised against expressing anger in a blatantly hostile, rude, smug, condescending, or sarcastic manner, as it tends to make the doctor less sympathetic and more inclined to disengage. Uncontrolled outbursts of anger can destroy the chances for a healthy doctor-patient relationship and erode necessary communication. Expressing angry feelings by yelling or offering insulting remarks tends to be counterproductive. A better alternative is to reflect on your reasons for feeling angry and then calmly discuss these issues with the doctor.

When anger is evident during a medical encounter, a doctor who is capable of a balanced response will not overreact or become defensive but will acknowledge the angry feelings, spend time listening patiently, try to sort out the problem, and offer solutions. You can tell the doctor is trying to do this when you hear statements such as, "I can see that you are angry; let's talk about it," or "I can certainly understand how frustrated you must be feeling."

It is appropriate for the doctor to acknowledge a mistake when your anger relates to an error on the doctor's part. There may be times when a person may come to believe that a mistake has been made when none has been made; it is important to listen to the doctor's explanation in such cases. Sometimes, there is a simple misunderstanding about the reasoning behind a line of questioning or medical strategy directed by the doctor. It is very useful to calmly inquire about these differences in understanding.

Controlling Style

While some of us want our doctors to take complete charge of the entire interview process, others among us find ourselves dominating the conversation, steering the conversation recurrently away from the issues the doctor is focusing on, and taking a lot of time, oblivious to reasonable time constraints and the other people waiting to be seen. Although this behavior may result from underlying anxiety about health or other reasonable explanation, it can greatly interfere with a healthy doctor-patient relationship. The doctor may feel manipulated and frustrated. An impatient doctor may openly express anger or begin arguing, but a good doctor will listen for awhile and then gently but firmly bring the conversation back to the areas that need to be covered. Sometimes, people who attempt to control the conversation ask the doctor personal questions about social relationships and may even behave in a seductive manner toward the doctor. In such cases, one should not be surprised if the doctor redirects the conversation back to the main points of the medical interview.

Denial

An individual who is in denial deals with a situation by refusing to acknowledge some painful aspect of reality that is apparent to others. This is a reaction that we all have in varying degrees when faced with the harsh reality of a significant symptom or medical problem. We attempt to protect ourselves from contemplating the potentially frightening implications of the problem by playing down the significance of the problem. Sometimes, acknowledging a symptom and talking a lot about it makes us feel we are showing weakness and that we are not strong enough to bear the problem. Unfortunately, denial can have grave consequences in this context. While one may think of oneself as a hero for ignoring symptoms, no doctor or family member will be handing out awards for failing to mention chest pain or shortness of breath that are symptomatic of an impending heart attack.

Some people may deny their feelings when they learn about a particular diagnosis, its treatment, or prognosis. Sometimes, in order to accomplish this form of denial, they may even appear overly chipper and optimistic in front of the doctor. It may be difficult to confront these feelings all at once, but health care providers should know what your reactions are and how you are coping with the problem. In some cases, such as severe depression, important interventions can be offered, including antidepressant medication.

A rushed doctor may be delighted to manage the care of a person who does not spend much time expressing problematic feelings, but a good doctor will recognize the curious lack of reaction where one would be expected and will try to probe gently for these emotions.

Dependent Style

We expect our health care providers to provide sensitivity, understanding, and empathy when we become acutely ill. On the extreme side of the spectrum, there are individuals who expect and demand extraordinary levels of care and attention over a limitless duration of time. Ironically, such individuals may idealize their doctors, who in turn find themselves making promises and trying to accommodate every wish of the patient. There may be great disappointment, and "the greatest doctor" can suddenly become "the worst doctor" in the patient's eyes when these expectations are not met. The best approach under these circumstances is for patient and doctor to establish a realistic set of goals that can be accomplished and discuss openly those that cannot be accomplished. The doctor will also need to be honest about the time he can devote to a problem and then work with the person to set priorities about what will be discussed during a given office visit.

On the other end of the dependency spectrum, some people are unusually passive or meek. Many people harbor an idealized image of the doctor as the all-knowing healer and father figure who will rescue us from medical danger. However, there are individuals who are completely passive in their care and too shy or intimidated by the doctor to give information or ask questions. Doctors will rarely complain about having such patients. Unfortunately, these people reduce the quality of their medical care by withholding crucial information, such as symptoms of concern and responses to treatment.

Depression

Feelings of depression are a common, yet neglected area of medical diagnosis and treatment. Depression may occur in response to loss or other upsetting life events, or dealing with a potential illness, and they sometimes indicate a major psychiatric disorder that can lead to suicide. A complete medical evaluation should delve into areas of psychological distress, including depression. Unfortunately, many evaluations fail to do so (see Chapter 8). If appropriate questions reveal symptoms of depression and there are signs of it, such as tearfulness, a lack of pleasure in life, difficulty sleeping, or changes in appetite, the doctor may ask further questions about depression. The doctor may also ask very specific question about suicidal thoughts, such as, "Have you ever thought about hurting yourself?" or "Did you have a specific plan for how you would do it?" Hopefully, the doctor will end such a conversation with a reassuring statement if the patient was actually having such thoughts. The doctor may also suggest a plan for how to deal with such thoughts should they recur. Referral to a psychological health professional should be considered for anyone who is having suicidal thoughts.

Nowadays, depression can be treated very successfully. It is unfortunate that the continuing stigma surrounding psychiatric illness has made many people reluctant to reveal their suffering.

The "Long-Suffering" Style

Some people tend to thrive on, and seem to be fixated on their feelings of constant suffering and their frustration with lack of progress in their medical condition, even if the reality is that their medical problem is under reasonable control. Such individuals usually have very little insight into the nature of their behavior and they are simply convinced that they are destined to have continuous bad luck. Attempts by health care providers to provide reassurance or assistance are usually rejected. There will be limits to the doctor's ability to reach such a patient; often, psychological consultations are needed to help the person deal with their distress.

Multiple Body Complaints

Some people suffer from multiple symptoms that cannot be explained, despite vigorous diagnostic testing and numerous evaluations. The symptoms may change from one moment to the next and fail to respond at all to medical therapy. In some cases, this may relate to inadequate evaluations or poorly understood diseases. However, there is a subset of individuals for whom symptoms are the manifestation of underlying psychological distress. Many doctors, unfortunately, do not appreciate the fact that regardless of the cause, these symptoms are experienced as real disability and should be treated as seriously as any other kind of illness. The body looks for ways to vent the feelings produced by extreme stress. Some people get an occasional headache or stomachache that is due to stress and others get more extreme and persistent symptoms. Doctors who tell their patients that "the problem is all in your head" are insensitive, and they miss the point that the pain is still real for the patient. These are extremely complex situations because the people who have these symptoms are usually very upset at the suggestion that any aspect of their pain may be psychiatric in nature, and because there may well be definitive physical components to stress or emotionally generated complaints.

Patients should not be put off by questions by the doctor about psychological health. It is appropriate and very important for the doctor not to miss possibly significant problems, such as severe depression or emotional trauma.

Overly Talkative Style

This book emphasizes the need for taking charge of your medical care and providing abundant information to the doctor, but we also emphasize the need for organizing that information and providing it within the time frame of the typical office visit. Problems occur when information is given to the doctor in a rambling fashion, in excessive detail, or it is not sufficiently related to the important issues. Doctors often perceive overly talkative people as being difficult to communicate with. Alternatively, an overly talkative style may be a manifestation of underlying anxiety.

Preparing medical information in the format described throughout this book should help keep the information that is conveyed focused. Doctors may occasionally redirect the conversation where appropriate but should never rudely interrupt the patient.

CHAPTER 29

Read This Before You Go to the Hospital

"The bedpan is a hundred-year-old contrivance that has, unfortunately, undergone few design changes during the century it has been used in hospitals. Doctors have not traditionally devoted long hours to analyzing or debating the phenomenon of the bedpan until they, as patients, are expected to use one. Then all hell breaks loose. However, after an appropriate interval of several months, we conveniently 'forget' how uncomfortable the device is and continue to insist that our patients be wedded to it.

I've often considered the old metal bedpan to have more esthetic than practical value. It seems to me that the cold, shallow, scalloped contrivance would be ideal for sliding on snow hills (like metal trays) or as containers for exotic houseplants."

PETER GOTT
No House Calls: Irreverent Notes on The Practice of Medicine

It is inconceivable. You were admitted to a hospital that carried an excellent reputation, yet you found that:

- The emergency room was crammed to capacity with people being examined in the hallways.

- Your calls for assistance using the call-button from your hospital bed often went unheeded.

- They brought you breakfast before a major surgical procedure when you were not supposed to eat after midnight.

- They could not reach the doctor to write orders for your pain medication.

- You were restricted to bed rest, but you could not get a bedpan for over an hour.

- There were roaches in the bathroom; the floor was filthy; and you could not get anyone to clean it up promptly.

- They forgot to give you your blood-thinning medication.

- You were supposed to be discharged, but no doctor showed up to write the discharge orders, and none of the doctors or nurses knew what was going on.

Sound like a stretch of the imagination worthy of a horror movie script? Unfortunately, this story did not require much creativity; all these experiences happened to the authors' family. Many hospitals are rated for mortality rates after cardiac surgery or for expertise in specific medical subspecialties, but perhaps rating systems should also be based on the time it takes for a call-buzzer to be answered, for bedpans to be brought, or for courtesy toward patients.

What can you do to advocate for your needs when you are admitted to the hospital? Although the intricacies of the hospital environment are worthy of an entire book itself, we offer a few suggestions here.

What to prepare before you go to the hospital:

- Bring the medical history forms included in this book if you have completed them.
- Bring your own medications to the hospital with you. This will be helpful when the doctors need to confirm the drug names and doses. The hospital may need to temporarily borrow from your supply in order to continue giving you the drug if your medication is an uncommon drug or is not on formulary. On the other hand, do not take your own pills without permission from the doctor because this can create confusion with the written orders, leading to an overdose or dangerous drug interactions.
- Bring a reasonable collection of personal items, including loose clothing, pajamas, slippers, toiletry items, books, or work-related items. It may be comforting to have a few family pictures or musical tapes/CDs with your favorite songs to listen to. Avoid electric razors or hairdryers, which may not be permitted.
- Bring cash for television service, magazines, assorted items from the gift shop, or if permitted, the cafeteria. Also bring insurance cards (see Chapter 25) and a list of contact information for friends, family members, your insurance company, and doctors. Avoid bringing valuable items, such as jewelry, that can be lost or stolen. If you want to have checks or credit cards available, ask a friend or family member to keep them for you.

What to do while you're in the hospital:

- Use the forms and advice given in earlier chapters to provide information and ask essential questions of the diverse health care providers you will encounter in the hospital. Write down all your questions and save them to ask your doctor.

- Designate your own personal advocates to be by your side as much as possible during your hospital stay. Your advocates can be close friends or family members, who should stagger the times they spend at the hospital in order to enable you to have at least one person with you for most of a 24-hour day. Getting a private duty nurse is optimal, but this can be quite expensive and many insurance plans will not cover it. Your advocate will be very useful for things such as going to the nursing station when your calls for urgent assistance are ignored.

- On the other hand, do not exhaust yourself by entertaining too many visitors. You will likely need a generous period of time to rest and recover from your illness.

Who's Who?

- Write down the names, dates, times, and content of what is said by anyone who comes to speak to you. For security and as a fundamental courtesy, anyone entering your room should introduce themselves and explain why they are there. Look for the hospital badge to confirm who you are dealing with.

- Observe whether the technician, nurse, or doctor has washed their hands before coming to see you. It is perfectly appropriate for you to ask if you are unsure.

- Take advantage of the time with your doctor and check that all necessary orders are written — for example, your pain medication orders are in place.

- Find out who will tell you about your test results and when you can expect to receive them. Try to get a sense of the schedule of events for each day.

- Beware of the "who's in charge" problem if you are admitted to the hospital. You may find that no specific doctor can convey a clear, overall picture of what is going on and what to expect if different doctors are involved in your care. Some medical or surgical services have nurse practitioners or doctor assistants performing day-to-day management and they may not answer to one specific doctor. It may not be clear who should be called to get information when you ask to speak to your doctor.

- Maintain a log of the names and contact information for each of the doctors who come in to see you. Clarify the role each doctor plays and insist on having *one* doctor who will take ultimate responsibility for communicating with other health care providers and who will take charge of your orders and discharge status. This is particularly important as the weekend approaches. Furthermore, if assistants, such as nurse practitioners are involved, make sure that they are not making crucial medical decisions without getting approval from your doctor. Contact your doctor directly if a doctor's assistant gives you a hard time about this.

Staff-Patient Relations:

- Treat hospital staff courteously and with dignity, and expect the same in return. If you like the care you receive from a particular staff member, show your appreciation by letting him know.

- Do not lose your cool if you are in conflict with a staff member. Express your concerns in a calm, neutral fashion and, if necessary, insist on discussing the matter with the hospital's patient relations representative or the hospital administrator. Discuss the problem with your doctor when she comes to see you on daily rounds.

Be a "back-seat driver" when it comes to your medications:

- Confirm the names and doses of medications each time you receive them and make sure that you are the person the medication was intended for (show the nurse the wristband with your name on it).

- If you do not know why a medication is being given, *ask*.

- If you suddenly receive a pill that looks different than those given on prior occasions, and you know your medication orders have not been changed, ask the nurse to check it.

- Make sure the drug you are being given is not related to one you are allergic to.

- Check with the nurse if you are due for a medication but have not received it. Be aware, however, that the exact time of administration of the medication may not be the exact time you took it at home.

- Make sure that it is okay to take your usual medications if you are scheduled for a special test or procedure. For example, it may be advisable to stop a blood thinner or anticlotting agent before a procedure is performed.

- Have your patient advocate ask these questions if you are unable to.

- Clarify the times when your medications are administered and see if the orders can be modified to avoid waking you up unnecessarily in the middle of the night to give you a drug. The same principle applies to timing of blood work or other testing.

- Ask your nurse when she anticipates completion of any intravenous medication you are receiving. Notify the nurse immediately when the IV is complete or if it appears to be working improperly.

Calling for assistance:

Consolidate your requests for assistance or information, if possible, rather than calling the nurses repeatedly for separate items. Use your discretion about asking for help. The reality is that many hospitals are severely understaffed. Try to prioritize your most urgent requests when the nurses are busy with emergencies, and defer your less emergent problems to when they are more available.

Designate yourself or one specific person to communicate with hospital staff, who can subsequently convey information to your family and friends. This is preferable to bombarding the doctor throughout the day with phone calls from different family members. Arrange a time for your doctor to communicate to that contact person each day about your progress and plans for testing and treatment.

Be persistent when it comes to getting adequate treatment for your pain or nausea (see Chapter 21). Many doctors are unfamiliar with the proper dosing of pain medications and often undermedicate out of an inappropriate fear of creating drug addiction. If available, request a consultation from a pain specialist or pain management service.

Ask your nurse to review your current standing orders with you. If they do not include medication for pain or nausea, and you anticipate these problems, request that the doctor write instructions for these medications to be given.

Do not be rushed to sign a consent form for a test or procedure. Use Form 17 in Chapter 22 to guide you in asking the important questions you need answered. The authors strongly suggest you consider getting a second opinion if you have concerns about a procedure and it can be delayed. It can be challenging to get an outside expert to see you in the hospital, but not impossible.

Be wary of eating before a scheduled test or procedure. Call the nurse and clarify this if you are suspicious of an error.

Insist on a clean room and speak to the hospital administrator or patient relations if hospital staff does not respond promptly.

Preparation for leaving the hospital:

- You should be informed of your discharge time a minimum of 24 hours before you are discharged. Discuss this with your doctor if you feel your discharge is premature.

- You can issue an appeal if your insurance company will not cover an additional day in the hospital.

- Ask your doctor what time you can expect to be discharged and who specifically will be coming to write the orders and when.

- If you anticipate being discharged, insist that you receive complete and information and instructions on necessary outpatient treatments, caring for a surgical wound, precautions related to an implanted medical device, dietary or activity restrictions, and follow-up care. Ensure that social service concerns are addressed, such as getting assistance from a home health-aide. Anticipate meeting a doctor, nurse, or social worker to review these items with you.

Here are some additional tips in case you need to visit an emergency room (ER):

- Make sure your own doctor knows you are going to the emergency room, ideally before you arrive there. Encourage the ER doctors to contact your primary doctor and confer with him about the best plan of action.

- You can anticipate being asked many questions about your past medical history, current medications, and allergies. Bring your completed patient information forms from this book.

- You may be hospitalized. Bring some of the personal items listed above if time permits.

- You may start your ER experience in the triage area, where your symptoms will be screened and ranked in priority of urgency. The triage nurse will decide whether the doctor needs to attend to you immediately or whether you can wait and what section of the ER you should be brought to.

- You may be seen in the registration area by a nurse or other assistant before you are seen by a doctor. Be prepared to show your insurance card and other billing-related information.

- Expect to wait a long time! You may sit for hours in the waiting room or actual emergency room waiting for individual members of the ER team to evaluate you. People with acute or more emergent problems will be seen ahead of you. However, if you perceive that your symptoms warrant more immediate attention than you are getting, insist on being seen by a doctor. Bring some personal items, such as a magazine or book to read while you endure the long wait if your condition is not severe.

- It may be necessary to repeat your story over and over again, especially if you are seen at a teaching hospital where medical students, interns, and residents, in addition to the usual nurses and attending doctors and consultants, may each ask for an account of your symptoms. Although this can be very tiresome, it does offer the possibility that one health care provider will pick up an important piece of information missed by another or may provide a valuable insight into your condition.

Example of a Completed History Form

The following are examples of completed Forms 2B, 3, 4, 5, 6A, 6B, and 6C, which can be used when seeing a new physician or a prior physician for a new problem.

Patient's Name: Mrs. Thorn
Medical symptom: *New headache for four hours.*

FORM 2B

History of Present Illness
Single Event

Timing and Circumstances:

Where were you when it came on?
At home.

What were you doing when it came on?
I was sitting in a chair, watching television.

When did it begin?
5pm today, 4 hours ago.

Were there any warning feelings that an episode was about to occur?
No.
Did the symptoms stop? If so, when? How long did the symptoms last?
Headache continued; did not stop.

Description:

List what you experienced step-by-step, from start to finish.
I suddenly developed intense pain in my head.

List what others observed step by step.
My husband said I looked like I was in extreme pain. He saw me having problems using my left hand.

If the symptoms stopped, what did you experience afterwards?
The pain never stopped.

Where is (was) the symptom located? (If applicable.)
All over my head but it was worse in the back of my head.

How does (did) the symptom feel?
It came on like an explosion of pain. It felt like a severe pressure.

How severe is (was) the symptom? (Rate from 1-10, 1 is least, 10 is worst.)
9 out of 10. I never experienced a headache as severe as this before. It was the worst headache of my life.

Are the symptoms getting worse, better, or have they stopped?
Staying the same.

Specify any associated symptoms?
I got very nauseous and vomited once. I felt weak in my left hand. I could not squeeze anything with my left hand.

Precipitants and Modifying Factors:

Is there anything that brings on the symptoms, such as lack of sleep or drinking alcohol?
No. It happened on its own. I was just sitting relaxing when it came on.

Was there any change in your medications, such as starting a medication or reducing a medication, when the episode began?
No.

Once the symptoms began, did anything make it worse?
No.

What did you do in response to having the symptoms?
I tried to go to sleep, but I couldn't fall asleep.

Anything tend to make the symptoms better?
I felt a little more comfortable sitting up rather than lying down.

Did anything you tried to make it better *not* work?
I took two Tylenol tablets. This didn't help at all.

Impact on Function:

How did the symptoms affect your functioning?
I couldn't squeeze anything with my left hand.

Were you disabled by the symptoms?
Yes.

How did the symptom affect your mood?
I got very upset and nervous.

If this is a longstanding problem, how did the symptoms affect your relationships, occupation, or home life?
The problem just recently happened.

Cause of Symptoms and Possible Fears About Them:

Did you receive a diagnosis for these symptoms?
Not yet.

What are your ideas about what may be causing the symptoms?
I have no idea.

What is your worst fear about what is causing the symptoms and the problems they create?
Could this be a brain tumor? Will I die?

Miscellaneous:

Have you have similar episodes in the past?
Never.

Did you witness or have you been directly exposed to anyone around you who has had similar symptoms?
No.

FORM 3

Past Medical History

History of birth and early development

Were there any difficulties in the pregnancy when your mother was pregnant with you?
No.

Was your birth full-term?
As far as I know.

Were you delivered with the use of forceps or cesarean section?
Not to my knowledge.

As far as you know, by what age were you walking?
Don't know specifics. I believe at the normally expected time.

By what age were you talking?
At a normal age.

Handedness:

Are you right- or left-handed?
Right-handed.

Allergies:

Do you have hay fever or specific bad reactions to foods or things in the environment?
Occasional allergies to pollen.

Summarize the names of any medications (including anesthesia) that have caused bad reactions, and list the details in the
Treatments form. Get itching from penicillin.

Pregnancy History:

How many times have you been pregnant?
Never.

How many pregnancies came to full term births?
Not applicable.

How many pregnancies came to premature births? Provide additional information:
Not applicable.

How many pregnancies were aborted? Provide additional information:
Not applicable.

Were these pregnancies spontaneous abortions, induced or elective?
Not applicable.

How many children are currently living?
Not applicable.

Did you have any specific complications or problems during any pregnancies? If so, provide details.
Not applicable.

Was labor induced or spontaneous?
Not applicable.

Were deliveries vaginal or cesarean; If cesarean why?
Not applicable.

Did you have any postpartum problems, such as infection or phlebitis?
Not applicable.

Were there any problems for the baby immediately after birth, such as jaundice or infections?
Not applicable.

Childhood Illnesses:

List your history of:

Measles?
Yes. As a child.

Rubella?
No. I had the vaccine.

Mumps?
Yes, as a child.

Whooping cough?
No.

Chicken-pox?
Yes.

Rheumatic fever?
No.

Scarlet fever?
No.

Polio?
No.

Other?
No.

Immunizations:

Type of Vaccine	Date or Age it was Last Received	Any Bad Reactions?
Tetanus	*I used to get these vaccines when I was younger. Last time I got one was over ten years ago.*	*A little sore on my arm where I got the shot*
Pertussis	*I don't know.*	
Diphtheria	*I don't know.*	
Polio	*As a child.*	*No.*
Measles	*I had the measles as a child, not the vaccine.*	

Rubella	*I don't know.*	
Mumps	*I had the mumps as a child, not the vaccine.*	
Influenza	*I had the vaccine each year over the past ten years.*	*Two years ago, I felt a feeling like having a cold one day after I got the vaccine.*
Hepatitis B	*No.*	
Haemophilus Influenzae	*No.*	
Pneumococcus	*No.*	
Lyme	*No.*	
Chicken Pox (Varicella)	*I had chicken pox as a child. I did not get a vaccine.*	*No.*
Other:		
Other:		
Other:		

Adult Illnesses:

List all of the illnesses you have had as an adult—for example, high blood pressure, diabetes, asthma, heart disease, cancer, HIV, tuberculosis, prior surgeries, psychiatric difficulties, accidents and injuries.
I have had none of these except for surgeries for my tonsils and my appendix.

Elaborate on specific problems by completing one of the following forms for each illness.

Specific Topics:

Name of the first problem:
Tonsils inflamed.

Date or age it originally began:
When I was seven years old.

How did it begin or present itself:
Sore throat.

Subsequently, what dates or ages did you experience recurrences or worsening or the problem?
Not applicable.

What were some landmark events during the course of the illness, what happened, and did it resolve?
Not applicable.

What were the names of physicians or medical centers where you were treated and the dates of any evaluations you received.
Don't know.

How was the problem diagnosed—for example, specific evaluation, examination, or test?
Don't know.

What was the diagnosis?
Tonsillitis.

What tests were performed? List the names of the tests, but fill in the details on the *Prior Tests Form.*
Don't know.

What were the most severe problems you experienced as a result of this illness?
Bad sore throat.

Currently, do you have any persistent complications/residual effects?
No.

Prior treatments: List the names, and list the details on the *Prior Treatments Form.*
Tonsils were removed.

Current treatments: List the names of your current treatments, but list the details on the *Current Treatments Form.*
None.

What is the current status of the illness? Do you have any persistent complications or residual effects?
No current problems.

What follow-up are you receiving and are any future treatments planned?
Not applicable.

Other comments: *None.*

Name of the second problem:
Appendicitis.

Date or age it originally began:
Age 13.

How did it begin or present itself:
Severe belly pain.

Subsequently, what dates or ages did you experience recurrences or worsening of the problem? What were some landmark events during the course of the illness, what happened, and did it resolve?
I developed bad stomachaches for two weeks. I had a high fever and my parents brought me to the hospital. They told my parents that it was lucky that they caught it in time because my "appendix had burst."

What were the names of physicians or medical centers where you were treated and the dates of any evaluations you received for this problem?
Age 13. It was some hospital in New York City. I don't have the specific name.

How was the problem diagnosed — specific evaluation, examination, or test?
Don't know. I remember they took some X-rays.

What was the diagnosis?
Appendicitis.

What tests were performed: List the names of the tests, but fill in the details on the *Prior Tests Form.*
X-ray of the belly.

What were the most severe problems you experienced as a result of this illness?
Very bad stomachaches. This went away after the surgery.

Currently, do you have any persistent complications or residual effects?
No.

Prior treatments: List the names, but list the details on the *Prior Treatments Form.*
They removed my appendix.

List the names of your current treatments, but list the details on the *Current Treatments Form.*
Not applicable.

What is the current status of the illness? Do you have any persistent complications or residual effects?
No problems.

What follow-up are you receiving and are any future treatments planned?
Not applicable.

Other comments:
No.

Name of the third problem:
Low back pain.

Date or age it originally began:
Ten years ago.

How did it begin or present itself:
I gradually began to have an ache in my lower back.

Subsequently, what dates or ages did you experience recurrences or worsening or the problem? What were some landmark events during the course of the illness, what happened, and did it resolve?
The back pain would come and go. It got better when I avoided lifting things but I still had it very often and went to see the doctor.

What were the names of physicians or medical centers where you were treated and the dates of any evaluations you received?
Dr. Tom Johnson. St. Joseph's Medical Center in Manhattan.

How was the problem diagnosed—for example, specific evaluation, examination, or test?
They did X-Rays and an MRI of my lower spine.

What was the diagnosis?
Arthritis of the spine.

What tests were performed: List the names of the tests, but fill in the details on the *Prior Tests Form.*
They did X-Rays and an MRI of my lower spine.

What were the most severe problems it caused?
Sometimes, I couldn't get out of bed easily. Sometimes the pain really limited my walking.

Currently, do you have any persistent complications or residual effects?
I only get very mild pains in that area once in a while.

Prior treatments: List the names, and list the details on the *Prior Treatments Form.*
Took ibuprofen and Percocet. I also was sent for physical therapy for several months.

Current treatments: List the names but list the details on the *Current Treatments Form.*
None.

What is the current status of the illness? Do you have any persistent complications or residual effects?
It mostly resolved. Very rarely, I experience a little pain in that area.

What follow-up are you receiving and are any future treatments planned?
I talk about it with my doctor during routine check-ups.

Other comments: *No.*

FORM 4

Family Medical History

Family Members

Include medical or psychiatric illnesses, striking physical characteristics, mental retardation, birth defects, miscarriages, or symptoms similar to ones you have experienced.

Relationship	If alive, current age	If deceased, age at time of death	Cause of death	Illnesses during lifetime	Age each illness began	Ethnicity
Mother		72	Stroke	Diverticulitis	60s	Irish
Father		70	Complications of Diabetes Mellitus. Had heart disease.	Problems from diabetes Poor circulation in legs.	50s	Irish
Sister #1	55			Irregular Heart Rhythm	50	Irish

Describe your ethnic background:
Irish

Extended Family Members

List other members of the extended family (grandparents, uncles, aunts, cousins, nieces, nephews) specifying if on father or mother's side.

Relationship	If alive, current age	If deceased, age at time of death	Cause of death	Illnesses during lifetime	Age each illness began	Ethnicity
Grandfather father's side		60	Possibly due to heart attack	Unknown	50s	Irish
Grandmother father's side		72	Breast Cancer	Unknown	60s	Irish
Grandfather mother's side		62	Cancer type unclear		60	Irish
Grandmother, mother's side		80	Alzheimer's Disease		75	Irish
				Arthritis	60s	

FORM 5

Prior Testing Results

Name of test: *MRI*

What part of the body was tested: *lower spine?*
Date of test: *About ten years ago.*

Where the test was performed:
St. Joseph's Medical Center in Manhattan

Results:
I was told it showed arthritis changes.

Name of test:
X-Rays

What part of the body was tested:
Lower spine?

Date of test:
About ten years ago.

Where the test was performed:
St. Joseph's Medical Center in Manhattan

Results:
I was told it showed arthritis changes.

Current Medication Treatments

Indicate the following for each medication you are currently taking:

Name of Medication:
None

(Other questions not applicable.)

Current Nonmedication Treatments:
None

(Other questions not applicable.)

Prior Medications and Other Treatments

Name of medication or treatment:
Ibuprofen

When was it started?
Ten years ago.

When was it stopped?
Ten years ago.

Why was it stopped?
Back pain got better.

Was it effective?
Helped a little.

What was the highest dose ever used?
Two pills every 6 hours.

Did it cause any side effects?
Sometimes I got an upset stomach. This got better if I took the pill with a meal.

Name of medication or treatment:
Percocet

When was it started?
Ten years ago.

When was it stopped?
Ten years ago.

Why was it stopped?
Back pain got better.

Was it effective?
Yes. It helped for about half of the day controlling the pain.

What was the highest dose ever used?
One pill every 8 hours.

Did it cause any side effects?
I sometimes got very drowsy.

FORM 7A

Your Psychosocial History

What kind of residence do you live in? (e.g. home, supervised facility)
My husband and I own our house.

Who do you live with?
My husband.

Are you single, married, divorced or separated?
Married.

Have you previously been married, divorced or separated?
No prior marriages or divorce.

Describe your most important current relationships?
Married.

What are some of the good and bad aspects of these relationships?
Happily married. We argue sometimes about my husband working too hard and not being home enough.

Have you been satisfied with sexual relationships?
Any difficulties in this area?
We are not very sexually active, often because we are so tired from our exhausting work schedules.

How has your medical problem impacted upon your activities of daily living, work, relationships and mood?
Medical problem just happened.

How are you coping with your medical problems?
It just happened.

Who is available to help you for emotional support, or if needed for transportation to physician, arranging financial needs?
My husband.

Important Experiences:

Where are you from originally?
Lived in the New York metropolitan area my entire life.

What is your highest level of education and where did you go to school?
Degree in accounting.

What do you do for recreation? What are your hobbies?
My husband and I like to play golf. We enjoy going to shows.

Where have you traveled in the past and when?
Seven years ago, we went on a cruise to the Caribbean.

Religion and Beliefs:

Do your religious beliefs affect how you allow yourself to be treated medically?
No restrictions.

Occupation Exposures Finances:

Are you employed?
Yes

What is your main source of income/support?
Combined incomes of my work and my husband's.

What have you been doing currently and in the past for a living?
I work as a senior accountant/bookkeeper in an airplane manufacturing firm.

If married, what does your spouse do for a living?
My husband is vice president in an investment firm.

How have you liked your work (the nature of the work, the hours, compensation, working with others)?
I enjoy it. It is very stimulating work but sometimes causes a lot of stress.

How would you describe your level of stress (physical and/or emotional) related to your work?
I sometimes get exhausted because the job carries a very high level of responsibility. A lot rides upon the quality of my work.

Is your work associated with significant risks for injuries or accidents?
No.

Has your work entailed any repetitive movements or major lifting?
Sometimes I get minor pains in my hands if I do a lot of nonstop typing.

Do you think any of your symptoms or medical problems are related to work?
No.

What have your work hours been like?
I get into the office at about 7:30 am, usually leave at 6:30 pm but occasionally have to stay till as late as 8:00 pm. I also sometimes work on Saturdays and often have to bring work home with me.

FORM 8

Current Health Form

Tobacco:

Do you use tobacco currently?
If so, do you smoke or chew tobacco?
No.

How much do you smoke per day?
None.

How long have you been a smoker?
Never.

If you do not use tobacco now, but were a former user, how long ago did you quit?
Not applicable.

How long were you using tobacco before you quit?
Not applicable.

Alcohol:

Do you drink alcohol currently?
Only rarely, socially.

How much do you drink in a given day or week?
Not applicable.

Have you ever had a drinking problem?
Never.

When was your last drink?
Do you have blackouts, seizures, injuries or other problems due to drinking?
Not applicable.

Have you had problems with work or relationships due to drinking?
Never.

Drug Use:

Do you use drugs illegally?
If so what types, how much and how often?
No.

How long have you been using illegal drugs?

Not applicable.

If you do not use illegal drugs currently but did in the past, how long ago did you quit?
Not applicable.

How long were you using illegal drugs before you quit?
Not applicable.

Exercise and Diet:

What kind of exercise do you perform?
No regular exercise. Occasionally go for long walks in the neighborhood. Sometimes play golf.

How often do you exercise and for how long have you been exercising?
As per above.

What does your typical diet consist of?
I try to avoid fatty foods. I have a pretty balanced diet.

Are there any restrictions in your diet?
I get stomachaches from greasy foods.

Do you use dietary supplements?
No.

How much caffeine do you consume per day?
I drink 1-2 cups of coffee per day.

Safety Measures:

Do you take the following precaution in activities of daily living:

Wear seatbelts?
Yes.

Bicycle helmet?
I don't ride a bicycle.

Sunblock?

Only when I go to the beach.

Is there a smoke and carbon monoxide detector in your home?

Yes. They are connected to our security alarm system.

Have you receiving the following screening tests?

Name of Test	Last Time Checked	Results
Tuberculin	*Long time ago. Cannot recall*	*I presume it was negative*
Cholesterol	*Six months ago.*	*Doctor said it was OK.*
Stool check for blood	*No but I had a screening colonoscopy (see below).*	
Electrocardiogram	*Six months ago.*	*Doctor said it was OK.*
Chest X-ray	*One year ago.*	*Normal.*
For women: Pap smear	*Not recently.*	
For women: Mammogram	*One year ago.*	*No abnormalities.*
Other:		

FORM 9

Review of Systems

Adapted in part from *Comprehensive History: Adult Patient.* In: Bickley LS, Hoekelman RA, eds. *Bates' Guide to Physical Examination and History Taking.* 7th ed. New York: Lippincott, 1999:35-39.

General:

What is your usual weight?

About 152 pounds.

Any recent changes in weight?

No.

Are you experiencing any weakness, fatigue or fever?

Weakness in my left hand.

Skin:

Any rashes, lumps, sores, itching, dryness, color change, or changes in hair or nails?
No.

Head:

Any headache, head injury, dizziness, lightheadedness?
Headache.

Eyes:

What is your vision like? Do you wear glasses or contact lenses?
With glasses I can see distances well. I also use reading glasses.

When was your last visual exam?
One year ago.

Any eye pain, redness, excessive tearing, double vision, blurred vision, spots, suspects, flashing lights, glaucoma, cataracts?
No.

Ears:

How is your hearing?
Good.

Any drainage from ears, ringing noises, spinning sensations?
No.

Nose and Sinuses:

Do you have frequent colds, nasal stuffiness, discharge, itching, hay fever, nose bleeds, or sinus trouble?
Occasional allergy to pollen.

Mouth and Throat:

What is the condition of your teeth and gums?
Have you had bleeding gums, mouth sores?
Good. No problems.

Have you had a sore tongue, dry mouth, frequent sore throats, hoarseness, or trouble swallowing?
No.

Do you have dentures, and if so, how well do they fit?
No.

When was the last dental examination?
About six months ago.

Neck:

Any lumps, swollen glands, goiter, pain or stiffness in the neck?
No.

Breasts:

Any lumps, pain or discomfort, nipple discharge?
Any bleeding, tenderness or swelling?
No.

Do you perform self-examinations?
Yes.

Respiratory:

Any cough, sputum and if so what color and how much?
No.

Any coughing up of blood, shortness of breath, wheezing, asthma, bronchitis, emphysema, pneumonia, tuberculosis, pleurisy?
No.

When was your last chest X-ray?
One year ago.

Heart:

Any heart trouble, high blood pressure, rheumatic fever, heart murmurs, chest pain or discomfort such as tightness, pressure or heaviness?
No.

Any palpitations, shortness of breath, shortness of breath upon sitting or standing erect, shortness of breath suddenly at night, swelling in your feet?
No.

Gastrointestinal:

How is your appetite?
Any trouble swallowing, heartburn, nausea, vomiting, regurgitation, belching, vomiting of blood, indigestion?
Good. No problems.

What is your frequency of bowel movements, and color of stool?
Twice a day. Brown.

Any problems with gas or cramps?
Any swelling, fullness of the belly?
No.

Any change in bowel habits, rectal bleeding or black tarry stools, hemorrhoids, constipation, diarrhea, abdominal pain, food intolerance, excessive belching or passing of gas, jaundice?
No.

Liver and Gallbladder:

Any liver or gallbladder trouble, jaundice (yellow skin or eyes), pale or white stools? Hepatitis?
No.

Urinary:

What is your frequency of urination?
Several times per day.

Do you have excessively frequent urination, the need to urinate in the middle of the night, burning or pain on urination, blood in the urine, urgency, a reduced force or caliber of the urinary stream, trouble starting, or stopping or holding the urine, dribbling, urinary infections, stones?
No.

Genital Male:

Do you have any hernias, discharge from or sores on the penis, pus or drip from the penis, painful or swollen testicles, history of sexually transmitted (venereal) diseases and the treatments?

What is your sexual preference?

Describe your level of sexual interest, function, satisfaction, birth control methods, condom use, and problems.

What is your exposure to HIV infection?

Genital Female:

At what age did you begin to have your period?
Age twelve.

How regular are the periods? What is their frequency and how long do they last? What is the amount of bleeding? Is there bleeding between periods, or after intercourse?
I underwent menopause in my late 40s.

When was your last menstrual period? Any pain during your period, pre-menstrual tension?
My late 40s.

Any vaginal discharge or itching?
Very rare itching. Not recently.

If applicable, at what age did you go into menopause and what were your menopausal symptoms? Did you have postmenopausal bleeding? If you were born before 1971, were you ever exposed to DES (diethylstilbestrol) due to your mother's use of this drug during pregnancy with you?
Late 40s. No postmenopausal bleeding. Never exposed to DES.

Any discharge, itching, sores, lumps, sexually transmitted diseases and treatments for this?
No.

Describe the number of pregnancies, the nature of the deliveries, the number of abortions (spontaneous and induced), and any complications from pregnancy.
None.

What birth control methods do you use?
Not applicable.

What is your sexual preference?
Heterosexual.

Describe your level of sexual interest, function, satisfaction, birth control methods, and problems.
See what I wrote in psychosocial section.

Any pain during sexual intercourse?
No

What is your exposure to HIV infection?
No exposure to HIV.

Peripheral Vascular:
Any pain in your calves during walking, leg cramps, varicose veins, past clots in the veins?
No.

Do you have cold hands or feet?
No.

Musculoskeletal:

Any muscle or joint pains, stiffness, arthritis, limitation of movement, neck or backache, arm or leg pains?
No.

If so, describe the location and the nature of the symptoms such as any swelling, redness, pain, tenderness, stiffness, weakness, or limitation of motion or activity).
Not applicable.

Neurologic:

Any fainting, blackouts, seizures, weakness, paralysis, numbness or loss of sensation, trouble speaking, trouble walking or with balance or coordination, tingling or "pins and needles", tremors or other involuntary movements?
Over the past few hours, I have had trouble using my left hand.

Any difficulty sleeping?
No.

Any problems with thinking or memory?
No.

Blood:

Any anemia, easy bruising or bleeding, past transfusions and any reactions to them?
No.

Are you recently unusually pale?
No.

Endocrine (Glands):

Any thyroid trouble, extreme discomfort from heat or cold, diabetes, excessive sweating, thirst, hunger, or urination?
No.

Are you feeling hot or cold all the time? Have you had unusual weight gain or weight loss?
No.

Any major change in your general appearance?
No.

Psychiatric:

Any nervousness, tension, depression or anxiety, memory difficulties, frequent bad dreams, frightening thoughts, feelings like others are out to get you or that others are controlling your thoughts?

No.

Common Medical Errors Related to Testing

Adapted with permission. *When Your Doctor Doesn't Know Best: Medical Mistakes that Even the Best Doctors Make—and How to Protect Yourself* by R.N. Podell and W. Proctor. New York: Simon & Schuster, 1995.

Organ System or Medical Topic	Problem
Heart	Neglectful prescribing and overseeing the use of anticoagulant or blood-thinning medication
	Relying only or mainly on total cholesterol measurements to prescribe cholesterol-lowering medications
	Under-treatment of patients with low levels of "good" HDL cholesterol
	Ignoring your triglyceride levels
	Ordering unnecessary invasive tests for heart disease
Gynecological	Your doctor says you shouldn't worry about a small hard spot in your breast because it hasn't shown up on any mammogram
	Your doctor tells you that because you've had one baseline mammogram before menopause there is no reason for you to have another mammogram until you are past menopause
	Your doctor sends you to an unqualified mammography center
	The technician fails to ask you if you have a silicone breast implant before giving you a mammogram
	Neglecting a Pap smear for very young or very old patients
	Your doctor fails to order a second Pap test after a normal first test, even though you are experiencing spotting or other symptoms between periods
	Endangering a woman's ability to have a successful pregnancy by not referring her for a colposcopy procedure after an abnormal Pap smear
Cancer	Relying only on a negative stool sample test in screening for colon and rectal cancer

	You are injured by a sigmoidoscopy or colonoscopy by an unskilled physician
	You aren't given a PSA blood test to check for prostate cancer
	You are a smoker and your doctor doesn't recommend a chest X-ray during your regular checkup
Abdominal Pain, Constipation or Diarrhea	Failing to do a urinalysis and blood count in evaluating lower abdominal distress
	Your doctor orders fancy tests for ordinary constipation
	Your doctor over-tests you for irritable bowel syndrome
	You are given an X-ray instead of an ultrasound test of your gallbladder
Respiratory	Your doctor prescribes theophylline for your asthma but fails to measure your blood levels of the drug
	Your doctor fails to order a tuberculosis test
Bones and Joints	Your doctor fails to recommend a bone density measurement to detect osteoporosis at the time you go through menopause
	Your doctor misinterprets Lyme disease test results
Endocrine System	Failing to do a blood test for thyroid function when the source of the problem can't otherwise be identified
	Your doctor fails to recognize that high blood sugar in the morning may result from too much insulin

Potential Causes of Commonly Encountered Symptoms

(Note, this is not a complete list of diagnoses and does not indicate which diagnoses are most common. Some serious causes are included in the list for the sake of being complete but may be very rare and highly unlikely.)

Symptom	Diagnosis
Amenorrhea	Pregnancy. Primary hormonal changes or imbalances or general body illnesses leading to hormone alteration. Tumor in the ovaries, adrenal glands, or brain regions responsible for hormone release.
Bleeding from rectum	Hemorrhoids, cancer, inflammation (e.g. ulcerative colitis), outgrowth (diverticulum), infections (e.g. parasites), fistula (abnormal channel connecting rectum to skin) of the intestines. Blood clotting problem.
Confusion or Memory Difficulties	Drug side effects. Stroke. Dementia, such as Alzheimer's Disease.
Cough	Problem of the breathing tubes (e.g. bronchitis, asthma). Problem in lung itself (e.g., pneumonia, blood clot). Allergies. Drug side effects. Lung irritants (e.g. smoking), Stomach acid backing up into the throat.
Dizziness or Vertigo	Low or high blood pressure. Drug side effects. Dehydration. Inner ear problem. Hyperventilation. Tumor, bleeding, or stroke in the brain. Anemia. Metabolic abnormalities. Anxiety. Impending faint.
Fatigue	Any stress on the body. Side effect of drugs or a special diet. Anemia. Infection or tumor somewhere in the body. Low blood pressure. Depression. Sleep disorder. Hormone imbalance. Eating problem.
Fever	Infection (e.g. viral, bacterial) anywhere in the body, allergic reaction to a drug, an autoimmune process, hyperactive thyroid.

Gastrointestinal Symptoms (Constipation or Diarrhea)	Drug side effect, overuse of laxatives, diverticulitis (infection of outpouching of intestine), cancerous growth in the abdomen, blockage of the intestines, irritable bowel syndrome, problem with absorbing food through the intestines.
High Blood Pressure	Essential (unknown cause) hypertension. Drug side effect. Excess salt in diet. Genetic cause. Stress. Blood vessel problem. Kidney disorder. Thyroid disease. Obesity. Insufficient exercise. Temporary increase when examined in the doctor's office.
Insomnia	Insufficient exercise. Too much caffeine. Depression or stress. Drug withdrawal. Sleep disorders like Obstructive Sleep Apnea or Restless Legs Syndrome. Breathing problem during sleep such as congestive heart failure or asthma.
Loss of consciousness, fainting or seizure	Transient reduced blood flow to the brain from a drop in blood pressure, heart problems (e.g., irregular heartbeat, heart valve problem, heart attack), blockage in blood vessels supplying the brain, dehydration, drop in blood pressure when erect, "vasovagal" attack (e.g. faint with extreme coughing, being frightened or straining when going to the bathroom), acute bleeding (e.g. bleeding per rectum). Gland problem. Drop in blood sugar. Hyperventilation. Bleeding or mass in the brain. Epileptic seizure.
Nausea or Vomiting	Problem in the abdomen or inner ear. Drug side effect. Stress. Drug or alcohol withdrawal. Pregnancy. Any illness in the body.
Pain in the Belly	Problem (inflammation, irritation, ulcer, tumor, blockage, distention, stones or bleeding) in any organ in the abdomen including stomach, pancreas, liver, gallbladder, intestines, appendix, kidneys, spleen. Problems of peritoneum (lining of abdomen), urinary tract or pelvic organs (e.g. ovaries, uterus), aorta (large blood vessel running through). Pregnancy or uterine lining (endometriosis) implanted outside the uterus. Esophagus problem. Heart attack.
Pain in the Chest	Problem with the heart (e.g. insufficient blood flow to heart-angina or heart attack). Heartburn. Hyperventilation. Musculoskeletal tenderness. Rib fracture. Problems of gastrointestinal tract (e.g. infection, blood clot, lung collapse)
Pain or Swelling in a Joint	"Wear and tear." Autoimmune process (e.g. rheumatoid arthritis). Drug effect. Infection. Abnormal deposits in a joint (e.g. gout). Joint injury.
Pain in Head or Face (Headache)	Mass or pressure (e.g. tumor, effects of high blood pressure, glaucoma). Migraine, blood vessel abnormality near brain

(e.g., malformed vessel, clotting, bleeding, inflammation such as temporal arteritis). Medication effect (including sometimes of medications designed to treat headache). Tension headache. Low pressure in head. Pinched nerve. Trigeminal Neuralgia. Infection in brain or fluid around brain. Dental disease. Neck problems. Eye strain. Psychological difficulties.

Pain in Neck, Upper or Lower Back	Tumor, infection, inflammation, slipped disc or blood clot affecting fluid, lining around or in the spinal cord. Problems of vertebrae (backbones), connective tissue between bones or muscles. Problems outside the spine such as the aorta, abdominal, or pelvic organs.
Palpitations	Anxiety, irregular heart beat, insufficient blood flow to heart, inflammation of heart muscle, too much caffeine, fever, low blood sugar, anemia, excess thyroid hormone.
Shortness of Breath	Problem affecting lung (e.g. infection, blood clot, obstruction, acute allergic reaction, asthma, bronchitis, emphysema, chest injury, lung collapse), heart (e.g., irregular heart rate, heart failure, inflammation of lining around heart), or chest wall muscles (neuromuscular diseases). Anxiety. Anemia. Thyroid abnormalities.
Sleepiness	Insufficient sleep at night. Breathing disorders during sleep (e.g. obstructive sleep apnea or restless legs syndrome.) Head injuries. Drug effects. Hormone problems. Depression. Anxiety. Not having enough time to sleep at night. Narcolepsy.
Swelling	Drug side effect. Backup of fluid (congestive heart failure, liver failure, pregnancy, inflammation, clot in a vein, cancers, or inflammation blocking the lymphatic system). Problems with water balance (e.g., drug side effects, kidney disorder). Injury, infection, or medical treatment on a limb. Standing or sitting for long duration. Menstrual period. Low protein level in the blood. Allergic reaction. Burn on the body.
Urination that Occurs Frequently	Effects of water pills, caffeine or alcohol. Inflammation, infection or anatomical abnormality in bladder, kidneys, or pelvic organs. Prostate problem. Pregnancy.
Weakness	Very nonspecific. If generalized weakness, has a similar differential diagnosis as fatigue. If a specific part of the body, could be a problem anywhere in the nervous system (e.g., brain, spinal cord, nerves, and muscles).
Weight Loss	Cancer. Diseases anywhere in body. HIV. AIDS. Tuberculosis.

Medication Categories

In the following list, we note categories of commonly prescribed drugs and suggested questions to ask your doctor about each medication.

(Questions in each section are adapted in part from *Classifications. Davis's Drug Guide for Nurses* by J.H. Deglin and A.H. Vallerand. Sixth Ed. Phila: F.A. Davis Company, 1999:C1-C60.)

Adrenergics: Medications that stimulate the release of chemicals adrenaline and noradrenaline, which dilate the bronchi (breathing tubes) in the lungs, stimulate heart rate, promote blood flow to the kidneys, cause blood vessels to become more narrow and increase blood pressure, close down the opening for urination, and dilate the pupils. (See bronchial dilators below.)

Analgesics: Pain relievers. Milder pain is usually treatable with non-narcotic analgesics; narcotic analgesics are used for more significant degrees of pain. Non-narcotic analgesics work by blocking chemical reactions that lead to a chemical that promotes inflammation and stimulates pain-perceiving nerves. Examples include aspirin, acetaminophen (Tylenol®), and a class of drugs called nonsteroidal anti-inflammatory drugs (NSAIDs), such as ibuprofen (Motrin® or Advil®), indomethacin (Indocin®), and naproxen (Naprosyn®).

Questions: Notify your doctor if you have a history of allergies to aspirin, bleeding disorder, peptic ulcer, liver disease, kidney disease, nasal polyps or are taking anti-clotting drugs, to see if it is safe to take this medication. Will this medication interfere with my other medications? Does this medication lead me to be at increased risk of bleeding at the time of surgery? Should I take it with food? Can I drink alcohol?

Narcotic analgesics (morphine and other opioids) reduce the mind's awareness of pain sensations. Examples include hydromorphone (Dilaudid®), meperidine (Demerol®), propoxyphene (Darvon®), methadone, morphine (MS Contin®), hydrocodone and acetaminophen (Vicodan®), oxycodone and acetaminophen (Percocet®), oxycodone and aspirin (Percodan®) and fentanyl (Duragesic®). A recently introduced family of analgesics is called COX-2 inhibitors, related to their interference with a specific segment of the conversion pathways of chemicals involved in generating pain responses. Examples are rofecoxib (Vioxx®) and celecoxib (Celebrex®).

Questions: Ask your doctor whether it is safe to take this drug if you have un-diagnosed abdominal pain, liver disease, history of being addicted to opioids, or recent head injury,. What other medications can I take, and which should I avoid while on this drug? How often can I take this medication? What activities should I avoid while on this drug? Can I drive or operate machinery? Should I avoid alcohol? Will I get dizzy on this medication? Will I become dependent on or addicted to this drug? Will I need progressively higher doses to get the same effect? How do I avoid getting constipated? Can I stop the medication at any time?

A class of analgesics used to treat migraine headaches is called "triptans". These include sumatriptan (Imitrex®), zolmitriptan (Zomig®), naratriptan (Amerge®), and rizatriptan (Maxalt®). An older form of treatment of the acute headache that should never be used in combination with the triptans is called an ergot derivative and includes dihydroergotamine and ergotamine (Cafergot®).

Questions: Ask your doctor if this drug is safe to use if you have a history of heart disease, liver disease, a type of migraine in which you develop weakness in a limb or other focal neurological problems (hemiplegic or basilar migraine), high blood pressure, are taking a medication called monoamine oxidase inhibitor, or are pregnant. If the headache doesn't go away with the first dose of the drug, how many times can I repeat it? What is the highest dose at any given time or over a 24-hour period I can take this medication? What other medications should I avoid while on this drug? Can I drink alcohol?

Antacids: Medications design to counter the increased stomach acid associated with heartburn symptoms (e.g. aluminum hydroxide, magnesium hydroxide).

Questions: Will this interfere with the absorption or dissolving of other medications I am taking? When should I take it with respect to meals or other medications? Are these safe to take in light of my other medical conditions?

Anti-acne agents: These drugs (e.g. isotretinoin; a derivative of Vitamin A) reduce facial acne by decreasing secretion of glands in the skin.

Anti-adrenergics: See antihypertensives and beta-blockers in this list.

Anti-anemics: These drugs combat anemia. One type is iron supplements, since iron is an important component of hemoglobin. (Keep iron supplements out of reach of children.) Alternatively, erythropoietin, a hormone that promotes the production of red blood cells, can be administered.

Questions: Will iron supplements interfere with the absorption of any drugs I am receiving? How should my anemia be monitored? Do I need my blood pressure monitored while on this drug? How much does this drug cost? How long will I require this medication?

Anti-anginals: These drugs treat angina (chest pain associated with decreased oxygen to the heart). One type of anti-anginals called nitrates (e.g. nitroglycerin under the tongue, isosorbide, or absorbable nitrate compounds) open up the arteries that supply the heart (coronary arteries) and thereby deliver more oxygen. (Keep an eye on expiration dates and don't store these in the bathroom.) Other types are calcium channel blockers (see below) and beta-blockers (see below).

Questions: How often can the sublingual nitroglycerin be taken, and at what point does the doctor need to be called? Can I drink alcohol when taking these medications? Should I be monitoring my pulse and blood pressure at home? Discuss potential drug interactions. (If you have diabetes mellitus, respiratory problems, or hypothyroidism, ask the doctor if these medications are safe to use.)

Anti-anxiety Drugs: Medications used to reduce nervousness and anxiety. Examples include drugs in the benzodiazepine class (e.g. clonazepam; Klonapin®). Another kind of anti-anxiety drug is called buspirone (BuSpar®).

Questions: Will I become addicted to this drug? What drugs should be avoided? Can I stop the medication at any time? How slowly should the drug be tapered off? Should I avoid alcohol?

Anti-arrhythmics: Medications used to control irregular heartbeats. These are categorized into different classes according to their mechanisms of action, which often involve regulating the flow of charged elements like sodium and calcium across the outer linings of cells. Class 1A and 1B are called "sodium channel blockers," Class II are beta-blockers (see below), III are drugs that extend the time of an electrical signal called the action potential (e.g. Amiodarone-Cardone®), and IV is termed calcium channel blockers (see below).

Questions: If you are elderly, or have liver or kidney disease, ask your doctor whether the medication dosage has been adjusted accordingly. Should I monitor my pulse and blood pressure at home? Can I take over-the-counter medications at home? What long-term side effects can occur? Will the drug interact with any other medication I am currently taking? Can I stop the medication at any time?

Anticholinergics: These drugs block the action of a chemical in the nervous system called acetylcholine. They may be used to reduce gastrointestinal spasm (e.g. dicyclomine; Bentyl®), treat peptic ulcers (e.g., propantheline; Pro-Banthine®), prevent motion sickness (e.g., scopolamine), reduce tremors (e.g.

benztropine; Cogentin®), and reduce urinary urgency (e.g., oxybutynin; Ditropan® or tolterodine; Detrol®).

Questions: If you have glaucoma, rapid heart rate, or myasthenia gravis, or if you are taking an antihistamine, antidepressant, or anti-arrhythmia drug, ask your doctor if you can take these medications. How do I deal with dry mouth caused by these medications? Will I get drowsy? Will it affect my vision? Will I have problems with urination? Will I get constipated?

Anticoagulants and Thrombolytics: Anticoagulants are anticlotting agents. Examples are heparin, or administered intravenously or under the skin (subcutaneously), enoxaparin (Lovenox®) given subcutaneously and warfarin (Coumadin®) taken orally. Side effects include risks of bleeding and other agents that block blood clotting such as aspirin may need to be avoided. Thrombolytic agents dissolve established clot in a blood vessel (e.g. streptokinase). Risks also include bleeding.

Anticoagulants should not be confused with antiplatelet agents (see NSAIDs listed under analgesics), which render platelets (the blood components responsible for clotting) less sticky. Examples include ticlopidine (Ticlid®), clopiogrel (Plavix®), and aspirin.

Questions: If you have a clotting disorder, ulcer, cancer, recent surgery, bleeding anywhere in the body or are pregnant, ask your doctor if it is safe to take this drug. What signs should I look for as indicators that I am taking too much medication? When should I notify the doctor? How often will we monitor labs to assess blood clotting? Should I take any precautions to reduce the chance of bleeding anywhere in my body? Are there any other medicines that will dangerously add to the anticlotting effect and should therefore be avoided? What diet should I be on to avoid interfering with the anticlotting effect?

Antidepressants: Medications used to reduce symptoms of depression. Tricyclic type include amitriptyline (Elavil®), desipramine (Norpramin®), doxepin (Sinequan®), imipramine (Tofranil®), maprotiline (Ludiomil®), nortriptyline (Aventyl®). Monoamine oxidase inhibitors include phenelzine (Nardil®). New classes of agents include selective serotonin reuptake inhibitors (SSRIs) such as fluoxetine (Prozac®), citalopram (Celexa®), sertraline (Zoloft®), and paroxetine (Paxil®). Venlafaxine (Effexor®) is a serotonin and norepinephrine reuptake inhibitor.

Questions: Discuss whether the drug is safe to use if you have heart disease, prostate enlargement, glaucoma, are pregnant or are breast feeding. What other drugs should be avoided because of dangerous drug interactions? Any specific foods that should be avoided because of potentially dangerous interactions?

Can I drink any alcohol? Will it cause drowsiness and will this interfere with activities such as driving? If the medication needs to be stopped, how gradually should this be done?

Antidiarrheals: Medications used to prevent or relieve diarrhea. Some agents work by increasing the bulk of the stool (e.g. Metamucil®) while others reduce intestinal movements (e.g. diphenoxylate and atropine).

Questions: Ask your doctor if it is safe to use this medication if you have severe liver disease, gall bladder disease or inflammatory bowel disease, are pregnant or breast feeding. Can the medication interfere with the absorption of other medicines I am taking? If diarrhea persists, at what point should I call the doctor? What other symptoms should lead me to notify the doctor?

Antiemetics: Medications designed to treat nausea and vomiting. Examples come from different classes of drug such as phenothiazines (e.g. prochlorperazine maleate), antihistamines (e.g. meclizine; see entry in this list) or anticholinergic (e.g. scopalamine; see entry in this list).

Questions: Will it cause drowsiness? Will I become dizzy when I stand up?

Antiepileptic drugs: Medications used to prevent or treat epileptic seizures. These are sometimes called anticonvulsants although not all seizures are convulsive (with shaking activity). Examples are phenytoin (Dilantin®), phenobarbital, carbamazepine (Tegretol®, Carbatrol®), oxcarbazepine (Trileptal®), valproate (Depakote®), ethosuximide (Zarontin®), gabapentin (Neurontin®), lamotrigine (Lamictal®), tiagabine (Gabatril®), topiramate (Topamax®), levatiracetam (Keppra®), and zonisamide (Zonegran®).

Questions: Will any of my other current medications interact with the antiepileptic drug? Can I drink any alcohol? Can the drug be used during pregnancy or during breast feeding? Will I need laboratory monitoring of the antiepileptic drug levels? What side effects should I notify the doctor about? What should I do if I miss a dose?

Antifungals: Medications that treat infections caused by a fungus. (See antiinfection agents below.)

Anti-gout agents: These agents reduce the pain and inflammation associated with the painful deposit of uric acid in joints of the body, such as the big toe. Examples of anti-inflammatory antigout agents are colchicine and indomethacin (Indocin®). Allopurinol (Zyloprim®) and probenecid reduce uric acid levels.

Questions: Can the medication cause crystals deposits in other parts of the body? Will these drugs have serious drug interactions with other medicines?

How much fluid should I have each day to reduce the chances of developing kidney stones? When should I take these medications with respect to meals?

Antihistamines: Medications used to block the chemical that activates allergic reactions or the symptoms of a cold. Examples include diphenhydramine (Benadryl®), and chlorpheniramine (Chlor-Trimeton®). More recently introduced, less sedating antihistamines include loratidine (Claritin®), cetirizine (Zyrtec®), and fexofenadine (Allegra®). Some antihistamines are used to combat itching (e.g., hydroxyzine; Atarax® or Vistaril®).

Another type of histamine blocker called a Histamine 2 antagonist blocks the secretion of acid in the stomach and is used to prevent or treat gastrointestinal ulcers. (See Anti-ulcer agents.)

Questions: Will these medications make me excessively drowsy? Can I mix this drug with the other medications I am on?

Antihypertensives: Medications that reduce blood pressure. Categories include drugs that work within the brain (e.g. clonidine; Catapress®), drugs reducing stimulating substances that normally exist in our body (reserpine), calcium channel blockers (see below), beta-blockers (see below), alpha-adrenergic blockers (see adrenergic above; e.g. prazosin) drugs that relax smooth muscles of blood vessels (e.g. hydralazine; Minipress), agents termed Angiotensin-converting enzyme (ACE) inhibitors which work by reducing the concentration of a substance called angiotensin II which tends to promote constriction of blood vessels. Examples are enalapril (Vasotec®), isinopril (Zestril®) or benazepril (Lotensin®). Diuretics (see below) and angiotensin receptor blockers (e.g. losartan; Cozaar® and valsartan; Diovan®) may also be considered.

Questions: How dangerous is it if I miss a dose or abruptly stop the medication altogether? Do I need potassium supplements? Should I monitor blood pressure and pulse at home? Am I at risk for fainting? Will it interact with other drugs such as cold remedies? Can I take it during pregnancy? What lab tests are required and how often?

Anti-infection agents: There are many classes of organisms responsible for infection. Antibacterial medications include Penicillin Class (e.g. penicillin, ampicillin), Cephalosporins (e.g. cefaclor; Ceclor®), Sulfonamides (sulfamethoxazole/trimethoprim; Bactrim), Tetracyclines (e.g. minocycline) Aminoglycosides (e.g. gentamycin), Quinolones (e.g. ciprofloxacin; Cipro®), and macrolydes (azithromax).

Questions: What are the signs of allergic reactions and when should I notify the doctor? If I am having gastrointestinal side effects such as diarrhea, what should I do? Do I need to complete the entire course of treatment? Can I sit in the sun? What drugs should I avoid while taking these medications?

Drugs used against organisms in tuberculosis include isoniazid, rifampin, and ethambutol.

Questions: Ask your doctor if it is safe to take these drugs if you have a history of liver disease, are pregnant or breast feeding, or had prior allergic reactions to ingredients of these medications. Do I need ophthalmology exams while on this drug? Should I take it with food? Will it change the color of my sweat, tears, saliva and urine?

Examples of antifungals include amphotericin, and fluconazole.

Questions: If you have kidney disease, ask your doctor if it is safe to use. How long will I need to remain on this therapy? Will it affect my blood counts?

Examples of antiviral medications include acyclovir, famciclovir, valacyclovir and amantadine.

Questions: Check with your doctor whether it is safe to take this medication if you have kidney disease. What side effects can I expect? Will this drug prevent viruses from being transmitted to others?

Drug used against parasitic organisms include those against amoeba illnesses (e.g. metronidazole; Flagyl®) and against worm-like parasites (e.g. mebendazole).

Anti-Inflammatories: Medications that reduce inflammation which occur as part of autoimmune diseases, infections, tumors, and other disease processes. (See corticosteroids. Also see NSAIDs listed under analgesics.)

Antilipemics: These agents reduce fat levels (cholesterol and triglycerides) in the blood. Examples of drugs that reduce cholesterol include lovastatin (Mevacor®), pravastatin (Pravachol®), fluvastatin (Lescol®), atorvastatin (Lipitor®) and simvastatin (Zocor®). Drugs that lower triglyceride include gemfibrozil (Lopid®).

Question: Ask your doctor if it is safe to take this medication if you are pregnant or breastfeeding. How often do I need to get liver function tests and monitoring of blood fat levels?

Antimanic agents: These drugs are used to treat symptoms of mania (a mental state of excitement with feelings of euphoria, irritability or grandeur that are out of touch with reality). Lithium is the classic agent but some of the anti-epileptic drugs such as valproic acid (Depakote®) and lamotrigine (Lamictal®) have also been found to be helpful.

Questions: What kind of blood test monitoring will I need while on these drugs? What are the side effects? What foods do I need to avoid?

Antineoplastics: Medications used to treat cancer. Drugs are either hormonal or agents that interfere with processes involved in different stages of the life cycle of individual cells, resulting in cell death of both normal and abnormal cancerous cells, but the latter are more vulnerable to the effects of antineoplastic agents. Examples of agents include alkylating agents which interfere with dividing DNA in cells (e.g. cyclophosphamide), antibiotic types which block the normal reading of information from DNA and RNA in cells (e.g. doxorubicin), antimetabolites which interfere with normal cell metabolic function (e.g. fluorouracil), and mitotic inhibitors which interfere with cell division (e.g. vincristine).

Questions: What precautions should I take to avoid getting an infection? What signs (e.g. bleeding or fever) should lead me to notify the doctor? Will I lose my hair? Should I check my mouth regularly for ulcers or redness? What should I do if they occur? Should I avoid getting any vaccines while on this medication? What foods should I avoid (e.g. can I eat salads)?

Antiparkinsonian agents: These drugs reduce the symptoms of Parkinson's disease (e.g. tremor, slowed movements). Since Parkinson's Disease and related disorders are associated with decreased levels of a brain chemical "Dopamine," these drugs either replenish dopamine or act like dopamine. Examples include carbidopa-levodopa (Sinemet®), bromocryptine (Parlodel®), pergolide (Permex®), pramipexole (Mirapex®) and ropinirole (Requip®).

Questions: Ask your doctor if it is safe to use if you have glaucoma, heart disease, obstruction in the stomach, or prostate enlargement. What medications should I avoid because of dangerous drug interactions? Should I monitor my blood pressure? Will it make me drowsy? Will it raise the risk of fainting? Will it cause me to get overheated? Will I get constipated? When should I notify the doctor about side effects I am experiencing?

Antipsychotics: Medications used to treat the symptoms of psychosis (severe mental illness with disconnection from reality and disorganized thought processes resulting in bizarre behavior, hallucinations, and delusions). An older term is *major tranquilizers*. Technical terms for the different classes of drugs include butyrophenones (e.g. haloperidol; Haldol) and phenothiazines (chlorpromazine; thorazine and thioridazine; Mellaril®). A more recent class of drugs termed the "atypical neuroleptics" or "novel antipsychotics" include drugs such as clozapine (Clozaril®, risperadone (Risperdal®), olanzepine (Zyprexa®), quietapine (Seroquel), and ziprasidone (Geodone®).

Questions: Should not be used or used with caution in the face of heart disease, glaucoma, pregnancy or breast feeding, diabetes, prostate enlargement, or gastrointestinal obstruction. Will it lower the threshold for having seizures? Will it cause fainting? Will it cause symptoms that look like Parkinson's disease? Will it cause abnormal movements?

Antipyretics: Medications to combat fever (e.g. acetaminophen, ibuprofen).

Questions: Ask your doctor whether it is safe if you have a bleeding disorder or ulcer. Can I use it in combination with other drugs I am taking? Should I take it with food? If the fever doesn't get better, when should I notify the doctor about this?

Antiretroviral agents: Drugs used to treat HIV infection.

Questions: What should I do if I miss a dose? What are the side effects?

Antitussives/expectorants: Antitussives are medications designed to reduce coughing. Expectorants and mucolytics are medications that help clear out mucus by changing its texture and stickiness. Codeine and dextromethorphan are examples of antitussives. Guaifenesin (Robitussin®) is an expectorant.

Questions: How long can I use this medication? If the cough persists, when should the doctor be notified? What other drugs should be avoided in combination with these medicines? Does it cause dizziness or drowsiness?

Anti-ulcer Agents: One type of anti-ulcer agent is a histamine blocker (see Antihistamines) called a histamine 2 antagonist, which blocks the secretion of acid in the stomach and is used to prevent or treat gastrointestinal ulcers. Examples include cimetidine (Tagamet®), famotidine (Pepcid®), nizatidine (Axid®), and ranitidine (Zantac®).

Another class of drugs is called the proton pump inhibitors and includes omeprazole (Prilosec®), lasoprazole (Prevacid®), pantoprazole (Protonix®), and rabeprazole (Aciphex®). Yet a third type of anti-ulcer drugs includes sucralfate (Carafate®).

Questions: Discuss whether the drug is safe to use if you have glaucoma, prostate enlargement, heart disease, thyroid disease with excess thyroid produced, liver disease, kidney disease, or are elderly. Can I drink alcohol? Does the drug interfere with any other medication I am taking? Will it make me drowsy? Will I have trouble with dry mouth?

Antivirals: Medications used to prevent or treat viral infections such as influenza. (See anti-infectives listed above.)

Barbiturates: A class of medications that facilitate going to sleep. Its major use is as antiepileptic medication. Examples are phenobarbital and primidone (Mysoline®).

Beta-Blockers: Medications that reduce stimulation by a part of the sympathetic nervous system on the heart, thereby reducing the heart rate and how hard the heart has to work. This in turn leads to a diminished need for oxygen. Beta-blockers are also used to treat angina, irregular heart rhythms, to reduce the chances of developing a heart attack, lower blood pressure, prevent migraine headaches, treat glaucoma, and decrease tremors (shaking movements in the limbs). Examples of beta-blockers are atenolol (Tenormin®), metoprolol (Lopressor® or Toprol®), nadolol (Corgard®), propranolol (Inderal®) and labetolol.

Questions: Check with your doctor whether it is safe to take the drug if you have heart failure, diabetes, liver disease, asthma or other respiratory diseases, slow heart rates, or heart block. Should I monitor my pulse and blood pressure at home? Will I get dizzy? Can I take over-the-counter treatments for colds?

Bronchodilators: Medications that open the breathing tubes in the lungs, reducing the shortness of breath occurring with breathing tube spasm in asthma. (See Adrenergics.) Examples include albuterol (Proventil® or Ventolin®), isoproterenol (Isuprel®), metaproterenol (Alupent®), montelukast (Singulair®), salmeterol (Serevent®) and terbutaline (Brethine®). Another type class of bronchodilators work by increasing the concentration of a chemical called cyclic-AMP and include aminophylline and theophylline (Theo-Dur®).

Questions: Ask your doctor whether is safe to take the drug if you have irregular heart rhythm. Can I combine it with over-the-counter cold medications? How do I use the inhaler properly?

Calcium Channel Blockers: Calcium channel blockers relax smooth muscle including that in blood vessels (thereby dilating them) and thereby improving blood supply and oxygen to the heart. They also decrease the oxygen demands of the heart by reducing the heart's force of contraction. Some calcium channel blockers can be used to treat irregular rhythms of the upper chambers (atria) of the heart. Calcium channel blockers include diltiazem (Cardizem®), nifedipine (Procardia®), and verapamil (Calan®).

Questions: Ask your doctor whether it is safe to take this drug if you have a history of liver disease, heart failure, heart block or uncontrolled heart rhythm irregularities. Should I monitor my pulse and blood pressure at home? (If on digoxin) will it interact with this drug? Can the medication be crushed or chewed? Can it be taken under the tongue? Can it cause dizziness or fainting episodes? Can it cause gum problems?

Cardiac Glycosides: These drugs stimulate the force of contraction of the heart, and can also be useful in preventing or treating some arrhythmias of the heart such as atrial fibrillation. The classic example of a cardiac glycoside is digoxin (Lanoxin®).

Questions: What are the signs I should look for of an excessive amount of drug in my system?

Cholinergics: These drugs increase the concentration or action of a chemical in the brain and nerve endings in the body called acetylcholine which acts on many body parts. Some uses include treatment of glaucoma (pilocarpine), to correct the deficiency in acetycholine action at the junction between nerve and muscle in the disease myasthenia gravis. An example is pyridostigmine (Mestinon®). In some urinary tract problems, it can help facilitate urination (e.g. bethanechol).

Drugs that increase acetylcholine in the brain may be used to reduce the mental decline of Alzheimer's disease. Examples are donepizil (Aricept®), rivastigmine (Exelon®) and galantamine (Reminyl®).

Questions: Ask your doctor whether this drug is safe for you if you have a condition with obstruction of urinary flow, asthma, peptic ulcer, heart disease, seizures, or hyperthyroidism-excess thyroid. If I have myasthenia gravis, how quickly will the medication work? What happens if the dose is too strong for me? When should I take the medication with respect to meals?

Cold remedies: Although there is no cure for the common cold, some medications can relieve some of the symptoms. Symptoms of nasal stuffiness for example, with "Adrenergic" agents (see above) such as phenylephrine (Neosynephrine®) and pseudoephedrine (Sudafed). Antihistamines are also often used. (See Antihistamines.)

Questions: What are some of the drug interactions I should be concerned about?

Corticosteroids: These drugs are useful when there is a deficiency of the natural body steroids or to reduce inflammation accompanying assorted medical conditions. They are similar to the natural steroids in our bodies that either control fluid balance or reduce inflammation. Examples include dexamethasone (Decadron®) and prednisone. Upper respiratory inflammations may be treated with steroid inhalers such as beclomethasone (Beconase®) or fluticasone (Flonase®).

Questions: Ask your doctor whether it is safe to take the drug if you have a serious infection, are pregnant or breastfeeding, or are about to receive a vaccine. If the medication is being discontinued, how fast can it be stopped? Will I need to take potassium supplements? Should I be on a special diet? Does it have any effects on the way my body looks? How long will I need this medication?

Decongestants: Medications that reduce stuffiness and swelling of the mucous membranes in the nose. (See adrenergics.)

Diuretics: Medications used to promote the elimination of fluids from the body through the kidneys. They are often used when there is swelling or backup of fluid due to heart failure. They may also be used to combat high blood pressure. Examples include "loop diuretics" furosemide (Lasix®), osmotic diuretic (mannitol), potassium-sparing agents (spironolactone) and thiazides (Hydrochlorothiazide®).

Questions: Ask your doctor whether it is safe for you to take the drug if you have liver disease, kidney disease, allergies to sulfonamide drugs, or are pregnant or breast feeding. When during the day should I take the medication? Should I monitor my pulse and blood pressure at home? What can I do to prevent dizziness or fainting upon standing? Do I need potassium supplements; how will we monitor how much I will need? Do I need to reduce my exposure to the sun? What does it mean if I get muscle weakness or muscle cramps? What over-the-counter medications should be avoided?

Hormones: (See thyroid below.) These agents replenish deficient natural hormones in the body. Examples are thyroid, steroid, estrogen, testosterone, insulin, and parathyroid hormone supplements. Estrogen is used to treat breast or prostate cancer, for birth control and to prevent osteoporosis. Progesterone is used to treat endometriosis (pockets of tissue from the uterus implanted outside the uterus), premenstrual syndrome and in combination with estrogens as a means of birth control.

Questions: What specific side effects should I be on the alert for? Will another medication make the birth control pill less effective?

Hypoglycemics: These medications lower abnormally elevated blood sugar in diabetes. Examples of oral hypoglycemic agents include chlorpropamide (Diabinese®), glipizide (Glucotrol®), glyburide (Micronase®; Diabeta®, or Glucovance®), tolbutamide (Orinase®), thiazolidinedione (Avandia®) and metformin (Glucophage®). When oral hypoglycemics are insufficient to control blood sugar, insulin injections are used.

Questions: Ask your doctor whether it is safe for you to take the drug if you have severe liver, kidney, heart, thyroid, other hormonal disorders, allergic reactions to sulfonamides or sulfonylureas, or are pregnant or breast feeding. Can I drink alcohol? What drugs do I need to avoid because they reduce or dangerously increase the effect of the hypoglycemic medication? What signs should I look for suggesting that my sugar level is dangerously low or high? Review monitoring of blood sugar and diet.

Immunosuppressives: Medications that reduce the body's defense against foreign tissues introduced into the body, such as transplanted organs and against itself in autoimmune illnesses. Examples are azathioprine (Imuran®) and cyclosporine (Sandimmune®).

Examples of drugs that modulate the immune response associated with multiple sclerosis include interferon beta-1a (Avonex® or Rebif®), interferon beta-1b (Betaseron®) and glatiramer acetate (Copaxone®).

Questions: What precautions should I take to avoid catching a contagious illness while on this drug? Can I receive a vaccination? What tests need to be performed regularly while I am on this medication?

Laxatives: Medications that help promote bowel movements. Some agents work by stimulating intestinal contractions, while others change the consistency of stool. Examples of stimulant laxatives include bisacodyl (Dulcolax®) and senna (Senokot®). Agents which increase the water content of stool include lactulose and magnesium citrate. Stool softeners include docusate sodium (Colace®) and bulk-forming laxatives include psyllium (Metamucil®) and methylcellulose (Citrucel®).

Questions: How long can I use this medication? Can I use it, if the constipation is associated with abdominal pain, nausea or fever? Will it interfere with the absorption of other medications I take? What time of day should I take it?

Muscle Relaxants: These medications relieve pain by theoretically reducing muscle spasm that accompanies some painful disorders (although the exact mechanism of action remains unclear). Examples are cyclobenzaprine (Flexeril®) and methocarbamol (Robaxin®). Some drugs are used to reduce a type of severely increased muscle tone called "spasticity" associated with neurological diseases such as multiple sclerosis or cerebral palsy. An example is baclofen (Lioresal®).

Questions: Can I drink alcohol while on this drug? What are other medications should be avoided? Will it cause drowsiness? If used for spasticity, will it prevent me from being able to stand up?

Pediculocides: These agents kill tiny insect organisms on the skin such as lice or scabies. Examples are permethrin and lindane.

Questions: What are the side effects with respect to the nervous system? Can it cause cancer?

Sedative-Hypnotics (Sleeping Drugs): These drugs are used to induce sleep before medical or surgical procedures, or to reduce anxiety. Commonly used agents include benzodiazepines such as lorazepam (Ativan®). Barbiturates (e.g. secobarbital) are less commonly used because they have more side effects.

Questions: Ask your doctor whether it is safe for you to take the drug if you have moderate liver, kidney or lung disease, or have a history of depression, prior drug addictions, or are elderly. Will I become dependent on or addicted to this drug? What drugs should be avoided? How slowly should the drug be tapered off?

Stimulants: These drugs are variants of amphetamines which tend to promote increased alertness in individuals with attention deficit hyperactivity disorder. Examples are methylphenidate (Ritalin® or Concerta®) or amphetamine and dextroamphetamine (Adderrall®). Some of these agents are used to treat narcolepsy, a disorder associated with recurrently going into a sleep state. Alternatively, a non-amphetamine treatment of narcolepsy is modafinil (Provigil®).

Questions: What side effects should I look out for? Can it cause weight loss, difficulty sleeping or change in my mood? Can it produce tics?

Thyroid Hormone Supplements: In conditions of low thyroid hormone output (hypothyroidism) these agents supplement the deficient thyroid production. A common example is levothyroxine (Synthroid®).

Questions: What signs should I be on the alert for that suggest excess amount in the body?

Thyroid Hormone Blockers: These medications are used in conditions of excess thyroid hormone production (hyperthyroidism) and work by either blocking the chemical reactions leading to thyroid hormone or with the thyroid hormone release. Examples are propylthiouracil (PTU), and sodium or potassium iodide.

Questions: How much iodine should there be in my diet? How should the thyroid response to the drug be monitored?

Tranquilizer: This is an older term that is not frequently used anymore. Minor tranquilizers are described under Anti-anxiety agents while major tranquilizer is an antiquated term for *antipsychotic* drugs (also listed).

Urogenital Agents for Men: Medications that treat enlargement of the prostate gland (prostate hypertrophy) include quinazoline (Cardura®), tamsulosin (Flomax®), and finasteride (Proscar®). Sildenafil (Viagra®) is used to treat erectile dysfunction.

Questions: Do my blood pressure or liver functions need to be checked regularly when on this drug? Could the treatments for prostate enlargement cause impotence?

Vitamins: Chemicals essential in small quantities for good health. Some vitamins are not manufactured by the body, but adequate quantities are present in a normal diet. People whose diets are inadequate or who have digestive tract or liver disorders may need to take supplementary vitamins.

Questions: What side effects can occur if I take too much?

References

(Note: footnote cites not included.)

Chapter 1: *Opportunities in Automotive Service Careers* by R.M. Weber. New York, 2002.

Chapter 2: *A Dream is a Wish Your Heart Makes: My Story by Annette Funicello.* New York: Hyperion, 1994.

Chapter 3: *As I Live and Breathe* by Jamie Weisman. New York: North Point Press, 2002.

Chapter 4: *The Encyclopedia of TV Game Shows* by D. Schwartz, S. Ryan, and F. Wostbrock. New York: Facts on File, 1995.

Chapter 5: *Past Imperfect* by Carol Daus. Santa Monica, CA: Santa Monica Press LLC, 1999.

Chapter 8:
Lucky Man: A Memoir by Michael J. Fox. New York: Hyperion, 2002.

When Your Doctor Does Not Know Best: Medical Mistakes that Even the Best Doctors Make and How to Protect Yourself by Richard N. Podell and William Proctor. New York: Simon & Schuster, 1995.

Chapter 9:
Patience for Patients by Mike Magee and Michael D'Antonio. In: *The Best Medicine.* New York, NY: St. Martin's Press, 1999:48-54.

Chapter 11: *My Stroke of Luck* by Kirk Douglas. New York: Harper Collins, 2002.

Chapter 12:
Anatomy of an Illness as Perceived by the Patient: Reflections on Healing and Re-generation by Norman Cousins. New York: W.W. Norton & Company, 1979.

Time on Fire; My Comedy of Terrors by Evan Handler. New York: Little, Brown and Company, 1996.

Chapter 13: *Living with Chronic Illness Days of Patience and Passion* by Cheri Register. New York: The Free Press, 1987.

Chapter 14: *Landing It: My Life On and Off the Ice* by Scott Hamilton. New York: Kensington Publishing Corp, 1999.

Chapter 16: *A Brilliant Madness: Living with Manic-Depressive Illness* by Patty Duke. New York: Bantam Books, 1992.

Chapter 17: *The Gift of Healing: A Legacy of Hope* by Beatrice C. Engstrand. New York: Wynwood Press, 1990.

Chapter 19: *It's Always Something* by Gilda Radner. New York: Simon and Schuster, 1989.

Chapter 20:
After All by Mary Tyler Moore. New York: G.P. Putnam's Sons, 1995.

Good Karma. The Best Medicine by Mike Magee and Michael D'Antonio. New York, NY: St. Martin's Press, 1999:152-159.

Chapter 21:
Headstrong: A Story of Conquests & Celebrations… Living Through Chemotherapy by Rena Blumberg. New York: Crown Publishers, Inc., 1982.

Chapter 22:
50 Years a Country Doctor by Hull Cook. Lincoln Nebraska: Nebraska Press, 1998.

Man to Man: Surviving Prostate Cancer by M. Korda. New York: Vintage Books, 1997.

Chapter 23:
The American Holistic Health Association Complete Guide to Alternative Medicine by W. Collinge. New York: Warner Books, 1996.

The Essentials of Complementary and Alternative Medicine by Wayne B. Jonas and Jeffrey S. Levin (Lippincott Williams & Wilkins; Phila. 1999).

Chapter 25:
In the Failing Light: A Memoir by David Tillman. Berkeley, Ca.: Creative Arts Book Company, 1999.

Health Insurance Resources: Options for People with a Chronic Disease by Dorothy E. Northrop and Stephen Cooper. New York: Demos Medical Publishing, 2003.

Chapter 26:
Cancer Schmancer by Fran Drescher. Warner Books. 2002. New York. pp. xiii-xiv.

The Mind/Body Connection by Erin Cardon. In: *My First Year as a Doctor: Real-World Stories from America's M.D.s,* Edited by M. Ramsdell. New York: Walker and Company, 1994:6-10.

Making Informed Medical Decisions: Where to Look and How to Use What You Find by N. Oster, L. Thomas, and D. Joseff. Cambridge: O'Reilly, 2000.

Chapter 27:

Anatomy of an Illness as Perceived by the Patient; Reflections on Healing and Regeneration by Norman Cousins. New York: W.W. Norton & Company, 1979.

Doctors and Patients: What We Feel About You by P.H. Berczeller. New York: Macmillan Publishing Company, 1994.

A Patient's Bill of Rights. American Hospital Association, Chicago, Illinois: 1992.

Chapter 28: *Flying Lessons: On the Wings of Parkinson's Disease* by J. Grady-Fitchett. New York: Tom Doherty Associates, Inc., 1998.

Chapter 29: *No House Call: Irreverent Notes on The Practice of Medicine* by Peter Gott. New York: Poseidon Press, 1986.

Appendix B: Adapted with permission. *When Your Doctor Doesn't Know Best: Medical Mistakes that Even the Best Doctors Make – and How to Protect Yourself* by R.N. Podell and W. Proctor. New York: Simon & Schuster, 1995.

Appendix D: *Classifications. Davis's Drug Guide for Nurses* by J.H. Deglin, A.H. Vallerand. Sixth Ed., Philadelphia: F.A. Davis Company, 1998; C1-C60.

Index

Note: **Boldface** numbers indicate forms.